D1435560

**Scientifically Proven to Reduce
Lines and Wrinkes by 34 Percent in Five Weeks!**

"Reading Dr. Howard Murad's guide to getting great skin . . .is like having a private consultation with the renowned L.A.-based dermatologist—only better."   —*Town & Country*

"Beauty from the inside out."   —*Allure*

"For a long time I have hoped Dr. Murad would write a book. His insight, his practice, and his peaceful nature are too wonderful not to share with the world."   —Cheryl Tiegs

"Offers an alternative to face-lifts . . . healthy doses of down-to-earth advice."   —*Seattle Post-Intelligencer*

"The book is packed with information that will change the way you . . . think about skin and give you the tools you need to make it look younger in just over a month. . . ."   —*American Salon*

"A straightforward self-help book that provides an easy-to-follow technique to slow down the aging process of skin. Readers will be surprised at how simple the 'Water Principle' approach is. . . ."
                                        —*Midwest Book Review*

"Dr. Murad is the Deepak Chopra of skin care."   —*Los Angeles*

WRINKLE FREE FOREVER

THE 5-MINUTE 5-WEEK

DERMATOLOGIST'S PROGRAM

Howard Murad, M.D.
with *Dianne Partie Lange*

ST. MARTIN'S GRIFFIN 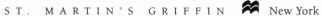 New York

WRINKLE-FREE FOREVER: THE 5-MINUTE 5-WEEK DERMATOLOGIST'S PROGRAM.
Copyright © 2003 by Howard Murad, M.D. All rights reserved.
Printed in the United States of America. No part of this book may be
reproduced in any manner whatsoever without written permission except in
the case of brief quotations embodied in critical articles or reviews. For information,
address St. Martin's Press, 175 Fifth Avenue, New York, N.Y. 10010.

www.stmartins.com

Interior illustrations by Stephen Sedam

Design by Patrice Fodero Sheridan

Library of Congress Cataloging-in-Publication Data

Murad, Howard.
    Wrinkle-free forever : the 5-minute 5-week dermatologist's program / Howard
Murad with Dianne Partie Lange.
        p. cm.
    ISBN 0-312-33106-1
    EAN 978-0312-33106-1
    1. Skin—Wrinkles—Prevention. 2. Skin—Care and hygiene. 3. Beauty, Personal.
I. Lange, Dianne. II. Title.

RL87.M873 2004
646.7'26—dc22

                                                          2004041881

First published in the United States by St. Martin's Press under the title *The Murad
Method: Wrinkle-Proof, Repair, and Renew Your Skin with the Proven 5-Week Program*

First St. Martin's Griffin Edition: May 2004

10   9   8   7   6   5   4   3   2   1

Discovery is seeing what everybody has seen,
and thinking what nobody else has thought.

Albert Szent-Györgi von Nagyrapolt,
1937 Nobel Laureate in Medicine

Contents

Foreword

Looking younger, staying healthy, being happy. These are the goals my patients have when they come to see me. As a practicing dermatologist for over thirty years, my approach with patients has always been different. I *know* that the results of aging skin have equally as much to do with a good skin care regimen and proper nutritional intake, as it does with one's emotional well-being. Whether treating celebrities or working mothers, my approach is the same. I believe that treating the "whole" person rather than just the skin is the key to my 5-week program.

During my press tour in New York City in spring 2002, it was my pleasure to appear on television shows such as NBC's *Today Show,* ABC's *The View,* and on CNN to talk about this book. The positive feedback I received was tremendous, and everyone seemed to want to know more about what makes my program so extraordinary. This response further validated the enormous need to explain how this method works, and to allow people the opportunity to adopt this program as part of their lives.

Why try this program? Because traditional skin care regimens and cosmetic procedures have failed to produce lasting results. They merely attempt to camouflage the visible signs of aging without actually improving the quality and health of the skin.

The program outlined in this book is easy to use, and, unlike any other anti-aging program, it is scientifically proven to not only reduce wrinkles and increase elasticity, but also to improve your overall health and well-being.

The key to this program's success is what I call "The Water Principle." Water is the anti-aging ingredient of the twenty-first century. "The Fountain of Youth," however is not found in a glass, or several daily glasses of water. In order to keep your skin and body young and healthy it is essential to maintain adequate water content in your cells. The main difference between aging skin and youthful skin is hydration. A baby's body weight is 75 percent water. An adult's is composed only of 50 percent water. The reason for this is that as we age, our cells break down and gradually lose the ability to absorb and lock in water. As this happens, we lose the smooth, firm, supple skin we once had.

Are you tired of wrinkles and roughness? Are you ready to get rid of loose, sun-damaged skin? Now you can do something about it. You may have to act your age, but your skin, your cells, and your spirit do not. I invite you to give me just five weeks and I guarantee that I will have you looking and feeling better, both physically and emotionally.

—Howard Murad, M.D.

WRINKLE FREE FOREVER

ONE

The Next Generation in Skin Care

You know the feeling. You look in the mirror and are shocked to see that the laugh lines at the corners of your eyes linger seconds longer than your smile. For a fleeting moment you can actually see the crow's-feet in your future. Maybe you're frustrated that the fine lines on your cheeks never give way to the precious ounces of costly creams you use every night.

By the time you celebrate your fortieth birthday, you may notice that the frown lines of disappointment and worry on your brow and the corners of your mouth have become permanent furrows. You might have picked up the habit of widening your eyes when you look in the mirror, trying to "lift" your descending upper lids. Perhaps you've made some attempts to approximate what a face-lift might do for you, tugging up on the skin over your cheekbones to see if the creases and folds on your face disappear.

If you've done your time in the sun, your mottled skin tone and sagging jawline make putting on foundation downright depressing. And, noticing that those scattered lines above your lips have become a feathery filigree doesn't do much to lift your spirits or improve your self-image.

For some men and women, awareness of these changes comes as a sudden surprise. "Did that happen while I was sleeping?" you wonder at your reflection in the toaster one morning. Or perhaps it was the off-guard glance as you passed by a store window that got your attention. "For a second, I thought I saw my mother," you may have confided to a friend.

I know about these reactions to the visible signs of aging because as a dermatologist who has cared for more than forty thousand men and women over thirty years, I've heard your stories. And too often I've seen the unfortunate results of hasty, desperate measures taken to turn back the clock. I've tried to erase the face-lift scars along the hairline of a woman embarassed by the red, ragged edges of the old incision that made her appear as if she were wearing a mask. I've seen how distraught a man can be when he learns that the pasty white skin tone that follows an overzealous peel cannot be reversed.

In skilled hands, most cosmetic surgery procedures either tighten or resurface skin without complications. But even when a quick fix is successful, a postoperative letdown isn't unusual. In fact, studies have shown that half of the people who have plastic surgery suffer from anxiety and depression afterward.

One reason for the letdown may be that while the person looks different, he or she doesn't necessarily appear any younger. The sagging may be gone, the fine wrinkles may be improved, but the skin still appears old and unhealthy. There's something about the new face that doesn't look normal. That's because no quick fix, no laser beam or surgeon's scalpel, changes the way the skin functions. Surgery to pull the skin tighter doesn't restore its youthfulness.

Reversing signs of aging *and* making skin more resilient and vital require treating it from the inside as well as the outside. This concept is the basis for the internal skin care that is an integral part of my program. Internal skin care repairs and rejuvenates. It *repairs* the supportive structures deep within the skin that give it support and elasticity. And, it *rejuvenates* the cellular machinery that produces fresh, new skin cells.

Dermatologists are skilled in using the tools of the trade to correct surface imperfections—the lasers and scalpels, and injections of botulinum toxin (Botox) and wrinkle fillers. But when patients ask me for the latest anti-aging procedure they've seen on the news or read about in a magazine, I ask them first to give me five weeks. That's how long studies have shown it takes for the benefits of my skin care program to begin becoming visible. Sometimes, I ask the esthetician in my office to give the patient a topical vitamin C infusion treatment before he or she leaves the office. The smoothness and brightness that occurs after only one fifteen-minute treatment usually convinces the person to try the five-week program. More often than not, when my patients see how much their skin improves without costly procedures or down time missed from their work and social life, they make a lifelong commitment to the program.

TAKE CARE OF YOURSELF, INSIDE AND OUT

The rate at which your skin ages, what signs appear and when, depends largely on how you care for yourself inside and out. The same steps you can take right now to begin making over your skin will also improve the health of your body. I include taking care of the body as part of my program because the skin and the body can't be separated any more than the mind and body can. After all, the skin is the body's largest organ, and it's the only visible reflection of the body's health.

My program is not complicated. In fact, most people are amazed at how quick and easy it is.

"Not counting the time I'm in the shower, the morning regimen takes less than five minutes," says Linda, a thirty-one-year-old marketing executive who has put her career on hold until her children, who are now eight, six, and two, are older. Her schedule-juggling resembles her days a busy executive, and she says she's become an expert in multitasking. "I clean my face as I shower. As soon as I step out of the tub, I spray my face with toner, apply the antioxidant renewal serum, and towel-dry my body and brush my teeth while the serum seeps in. Then I moisturize. Swallow the supplements and, boom, I'm finished and out the door."

Linda keeps sunscreen in the car and applies it liberally, rain or shine, while the children are buckling up and settling in for the ride to school. (They've already learned to put on sunscreen after washing their faces.) "The morning steps have become a habit that I don't even think about," she says.

At night, Linda completes her evening regimen soon after dinner, so if she falls asleep while reading to her children, as she often does, there's no chance of missing the second part of the daily program.

Every month, Linda has a vitamin C infusion facial at my day spa to further nourish her skin with antioxidants. These salon treatments also give her an hour to herself. The relaxation of being pampered helps her skin, too. As I'll explain in chapter 14, I'm convinced that relaxation and being touched during a massage or a facial are essential antidotes to the cascading side effects of stress on the skin.

There is no single procedure, not even a deep face-lift or peel, or a single ingredient, not even my favorite antioxidant and sun protector, pomegranate, that will reverse all the aging changes etched on your face. What does work is a complete, holistic program that addresses all the causes of those changes. Also, by restoring the skin's internal environment, all of the skin's layers—from the deepest layer of fat to the topmost layer of skin cells—are fully hydrated and protected from further damage.

In nourishing, repairing, and protecting your skin, you will also be restoring health to your body. Think about it. The cells of your vital organs, like those of your skin, need a constant supply of oxygen, water, and nutrients. The cells of your heart, liver, brain, and skin have similar needs, which I don't believe can be provided by the food that most of us eat.

In repairing and rejuvenating the connective tissue that makes your skin resilient, for instance, this program also encourages the health of connective tissue in blood vessels, nerves, tendons, and joints. Curtailing inflammation in the skin also diminishes inflammation in the blood vessels that supply the heart and the brain. And every cell needs to be well hydrated in order to perform. That's why I think it's so important to take hydrating supplements such as fatty acids.

AN INCLUSIVE PROGRAM

The anti-aging program I've developed is an *inclusive* program. By inclusive I mean that the program includes

- treating the surface signs of aging that bother you
- enriching the body internally with the materials needed to maintain a healthy water balance, stimulate new cell growth, and repair vital skin structures
- reducing the influences of negative emotions and stress on the skin and body

Clinical studies have shown that each step of my program has its unique, measurable benefits, and I'll be describing the results of that research in the following chapters. The daily regimens combine what you need to do in the morning and the evening in an easy-to-follow format. The products in the regimens are those that

I prescribe to my patients, use in my spa, and distribute to estheticians throughout the country. Because I've designed these formulations and tested them, I'm certain that they will work for you. However, to give you choices, I've included alternative products that contain a similar recipe and are also widely available. In the appendix, you will find a list of the key ingredients in those products. Cosmetic companies do not share their product formulations, and while products may contain the same ingredients, they are not identical and the amounts can vary considerably. How the ingredients are combined is important, too. You may have to do some experimenting to find the substitution that works best for you.

I have also designed and patented supplements that contain the necessary nutrients in the amounts that I have found most effective and that are safe. However, if you prefer to assemble your own favorite brands of formulas, I have provided a breakdown of the ingredients in my formulas. Keep in mind, though, that supplements are not regulated as drugs are, so different brands may vary in quality. I suggest you stick with known brands. Also, if you have any health conditions or are on any medications, check with your personal physician before taking any supplement, since there may be interactions that could be harmful.

By following my program, you will turn back the clock in a natural way. One part of the program assists in repairing collagen. One boosts hydration. Another part focuses on sun protection. These steps also work synergistically, meaning the combination of steps in the program is more effective than each single step alone.

To achieve what I call an *ageless* face, a face that is youthful and natural yet has definition and character, all you have to do is follow a simple morning and evening regimen, eat a skin-healthy diet, and take some time out to relax. But as simple as my program is, some people may be tempted to take short cuts, especially when it comes to taking time out for a facial or to eat in a more healthful way. It's true that if you've relied on fast food and frozen prepared entrées, shopping and preparing fresh food takes time. In my experience most people get more efficient at it, and you'll look and feel so much better that the time investment will be worthwhile. If you're tempted to skip a step, think about this: Isn't it time you take care of yourself as well as you care for others?

HOW MY PROGRAM EVOLVED

Scientific breakthroughs are rarely sudden, and skin care discoveries are no exception. These advances come as a result of uncovering one piece of the aging skin puzzle and putting it together with another over many years. The new theory must be tested in the laboratory and then in humans. Researchers must then prove that the results are consistent and reproducible, and that the ingredient or product that helps treat the skin is safe for most people.

This painstaking process is not done by one person in one laboratory, but by scientists all over the world. We meet and share the results of our efforts and question each other's work frequently. We publish the results of our tests and talk about them at scientific meetings. A discovery by a researcher in Berlin may be the missing piece a physician in Los Angeles has been searching for. That's the way science works.

I'm telling you this because I think it's important to appreciate the years of study, experimentation, and testing by others and myself that have culminated in the program I'm going to share with you. The evolution of my inclusive skin care program mirrors the cutting edge of several important advances in skin physiology, nutrition, and psychology.

An example is the fairly recent awareness that stress directly affects skin. Throughout my years of medical practice, I've seen the impact of stress and the havoc that hormones released as a result can create. And I've seen how some people's skin improves when they add some form of emotional self-care to the treatments I prescribe.

Just last year, researchers at the University of Dresden in Germany made an important discovery that may help explain what other dermatologists and I have observed. The German scientists found that a particular stress hormone fits like a key into the lock of receptor in the skin and causes damaging inflammation, the kind that leads to wrinkles and hair loss. Another piece of the puzzle, linking stress and skin function, has been found.

I began devising my skin care program in 1972, as I was completing my residency at the University of California at Los Angeles. At that time, I was like most dermatologists in believing that my job was to treat skin disease. Yet soon after I started my private practice, it became clear to me that many of my patients were complaining of what medical professionals considered "cosmetic" problems. These men and women not only had psoriasis, they had wrinkles, too. Yes, they had acne, but melasma, or hyperpigmentation, that created dark blotches on their complexion, also troubled them. Rather than ignore the "cosmetic" problems that were causing my patients so much distress, I gave them my full attention. At the time, this was an enormous leap in medicine.

In 1984 I became one of the first dermatologists to invite an esthetician to join my practice. I shared with her my knowledge of how healthy skin functions and how it needs to be treated, and she shared with me her years of experience in deep cleansing, moisturizing, and massaging the skin. I began to realize that being touched and cared for, which is what happens in the hands of a good esthetician, relieves stress and helps people feel better about themselves. I saw that taking care of one's self is healing medicine, too.

I opened A Sense of Self skin care spa in 1987 in Brentwood, a Los Angeles community. It was one of the first day spas to integrate health and beauty into what I called an *Optimal Health Care* program. In addition to medically oriented skin care, clients could consult with a nutritionist, a fitness trainer, and have treatment facials by a trained esthetician.

Before I became a medical doctor, I was a pharmacist, and in the 1970s I began working with a cosmetic chemist to design unique treatments and products that met my patients' individual needs. In 1990, I made the now ubiquitous alpha hydroxy acids (AHAs) available to the public. Alpha hydroxy acids speed up the skin's natural shedding process. By removing the dead, dry cells from the surface of the skin, moisturizing products can be more easily absorbed, and the skin immediately becomes smoother. Alpha hydroxy acids remain an important part of my program for most skin types, and you'll be learning more about them later in this book.

Initially, the formulas I developed were only available to patients in my care. Then, my experience using AHAs in thousands of patients and spa clients and seeing how exfoliation improved their skin convinced me to formulate a line of AHA-based products. In 1990 I introduced AHAs to the professional skin care industry with home care products and the AHA Rapid Exfoliator Professional Treatment, both of which are now standard treatments. With AHAs, "feel good" facials became true treatment facials.

COSMETICS GET SERIOUS

Products with AHAs are included in a category of skin treatment products called *cosmeceuticals,* a term introduced twenty years ago by dermatologist Albert M. Kligman to describe agents applied to the skin that are more active than cosmetics but not so active that they have uncomfortable or harmful side effects, as drugs do. Cosmeceuticals have been medically defined as "product[s] with an activity that is *intended* to treat or prevent a (mild) skin (abnormality)." Although the Food and Drug Administration (FDA) has not officially recognized cosmeceuticals and doesn't regulate them, other countries have acknowledged that some cosmetic ingredients have a biological effect on skin. In Japan, for example, these active ingredients are called "quasidrugs" and must be proven mild and safe.

Several of the ingredients I'm going to suggest you look for are in cosmeceutical products. However, keep in mind that since the FDA does not regulate these products, the activity of the ingredients will vary. You'll need to pay close attention to how your skin reacts to them, and perhaps modify your regimen to suit your own skin.

FEEDING THE SKIN

Skin is a responsive, active organ. In a sense, it's a factory, because it continually maintains its own supporting structures and manufactures skin cells and the gel-like material that holds them together.

Whatever goes into the body affects how the organs function. So if you want healthy skin, you have to supply it with the necessary building blocks for cell membranes and connective tissue. These include proteins or amino acids; water-bonding elements such as phospholipids; fatty acids; lecithin, vitamins B and C; and trace minerals.

The concept behind my program is that as this skin cell factory ages, it becomes less efficient. (There are several theories for this decline in efficiency—or aging—which are discussed in chapter 6.) I have found that by increasing the supply of raw materials—protective and reparative agents—the factory can resume normal, more youthful production.

This concept is also the basis for the rapidly developing field of *nutraceuticals.* Nutraceuticals are nutrients that act like pharmaceuticals to prevent or treat chronic conditions and disease. When it comes to aging skin, nutraceuticals are one more means to replenish the skin cell factory. I began recommending nutraceuticals in the 1980's and became especially partial to pomegranate extract. It is a powerful natural antioxidant, and after my research confirmed it could boost the effectiveness of sunscreen, I began including it in sunscreens and supplements in 2000.

Because the skin is such an efficient barrier, and its upper layer has no blood supply, it's difficult to get nutrients and other vital materials from the skin's surface down into the deeper layers of the epidermis, where the cells are nourished. By seeing what could be accomplished with nutraceuticals in other health conditions, it became clear to me that supplements—nourishing the skin from within, from the bloodstream—could make up for deficiencies in the skin.

Now scientists are on the cutting edge of *techniceuticals,* a term I coined for enhancing new technologies with other agents. Along with laser resurfacing, for instance, I use vitamin C infusions and nutritional supplements to directly restore nutrients to the dermis. With infusion technology, for example, it is possible to deliver antioxidants, anti-inflammatory agents, hydrating chemicals, and collagen-building materials directly to the dermis. For the last two years, I have been using the infusion technique to flood the skin with high concentrations of vitamin C with excellent results that you will learn about in chapter 11.

A DIFFERENCE YOU CAN SEE

Some improvements, such as the glow that comes from removing dead, dry skin cells and improving circulation to the skin will be noticeable immediately. Other, more dramatic changes—diminished fine lines, fading of hyperpigmented areas, increased production of collagen—will begin to appear in about five weeks. And the improvement will continue as long as you follow the program. Finally, some age-related changes are prevented entirely. Consistent use of the anti-aging supplements and sun protection means you'll never see what might have happened had you continued to ignore your skin's needs for hydration, repair, and protection.

My program has evolved over nearly three decades and encompasses five principles of skin care.

- First, the skin must be healthy. Its most important function is to serve as a barrier to hold moisture in and keep irritants, toxins, and invaders out. And it can only perform these tasks if it's healthy.
- Second, supply the skin with water inside and out and protect and repair the cell membranes so that each and every cell of the body is filled to its maximum capacity with water. Everything done for the skin is directed toward boosting its water supply.
- Third, repair any damage that has occurred as a result of the external and internal insults on a daily basis. By restoring and maintaining the skin's health, it begins to function more youthfully.
- Fourth, skin must be protected from further environmental injury as well as damage from internal forces, like stress.
- Fifth, accomplish all of the above objectives with an *inclusive* program of a variety of ingredients and supplements that target all the causes of aging, not just one. Everything done to and for the skin is based on a recipe of antioxidants, anti-inflammatory agents, hydrators, collagen-builders, and protectors. No single product or ingredient

can do everything that has to be done to repair and rejuvenate skin.

The processes that cause aging can't be permanently stopped. But I've seen that aging of the skin can be slowed and much of the damage can be repaired. To achieve this you have to follow all the steps of the program consistently. Even the effects of a potent drug such as Retin-A, which improves fine lines and stimulates collagen production, doesn't last indefinitely. Studies have shown that the skin reverts to its pretreatment state once the drug is stopped.

Cell turnover and collagen production are ongoing physiologic processes that have to be maintained at their optimal level. I believe this can be done by continuously feeding the skin with nutrients that repair, restore, and protect it.

The cosmeceuticals and nutraceuticals that are the foundation of my anti-aging program are the results of research efforts of many scientists over the past decade. In some cases, these natural, active ingredients, such as vitamin C, are not new, but the technology is now available to incorporate them into products that are stable and pleasant to use. Some ingredients, such as hydroxy acids, have simply been rediscovered and are now in formulas that are gentle and suitable for all skin types.

Skin treatment products are now widely available that include powerful antioxidants to counter the free radicals that are partly the result of the aging process and partly the result of environmental insults. These products also include anti-inflammatory agents that soothe the skin. And finally, some are superhydrating agents that attract water to the skin and improve its ability to hold on to water.

There are supplements that restore health and vitality to the skin cells and are beneficial to all the cells of the body. After all, free radical damage doesn't just affect the skin, it affects the walls of blood vessels and lung and brain tissue. Every cell in the body is susceptible. Indeed, scientists are now learning that inflammation plays a critical role in the development of many of the diseases of aging such as diabetes, heart disease, and cancer.

Which brings us back to my basic premise for healthy skin care. Whatever you do for the health of your skin will improve the health of your body. Whatever you do for the health of your body will improve the health—and appearance—of your skin. My philosophy can be summed up simply: Make your skin healthy, and your body will follow.

THE BASICS

You're already doing some variation of basic skin care. You're washing your face every morning and night. Possibly you're doing some kind of exfoliation with a hydroxy acid, a facial scrub, or a loofah-like sponge or cloth. (Men give themselves an exfoliating treatment every time they shave.) It's likely that you're following your cleansing with a moisturizer. And, if you're smart you top this off with sun protection. But are you performing these basic steps with the least amount of damage to your skin? Inflammation, which can be caused by using irritating products, is one of the major causes of dryness and wrinkling. And are you making the most of your basic skin care regimen to infuse your skin with nutrients and natural moisturizers?

Daily skin care with products that include my basic recipe of ingredients, which you'll soon learn about, is your first defense against aging. If the barrier function of your skin is compromised in any way, it can't do its protective job.

When I talk with patients in my practice, I never assume that they already do what's best for their skin type, and I'm not going to assume that readers do either. So please don't skip the descriptions of the skin care steps, even if you think you already have the basics down pat.

ENVIRONMENTAL AGING

For decades skin researchers have made a distinction between intrinsic and extrinsic aging. Skin, like every other organ in your body, begins to age when you are about twenty as a result of internal cellular changes, many of which are genetically preprogrammed. But skin is different from other organs in that it is also exposed to external injury, mainly environmental damage by sunlight and pollution. Environmental factors also include those things we do to ourselves, such as eating poorly, drinking too much alcohol, smoking, and taking certain medications. These environmental factors cause biological changes that accelerate the natural intrinsic aging process.

It's been estimated that 80 to 90 percent of the visible signs of aging are caused by environmental injury, and that the remaining 20 percent are due to internal aging factors that we once thought to be beyond our influence. I've done an exhaustive search of the literature and haven't been able to find the source of this famously high percentage, but I do think it's safe to assume that much of the damage we see as aging is the result of injury from the outside—that is, overexposure to the sun and pollutants in the atmosphere.

When I was in medical school, my dermatology professor taught us to understand the difference between extrinsic and intrinsic aging by saying, "Just look at the backs of your hands. What you see is the result of external, or extrinsic, aging. Now look at the inside of your wrist. The changes you see there are the result of intrinsic aging."

Where I differ from the party line on extrinsic and intrinsic aging is that I don't believe in a simple division into inside and outside factors. Rather I believe these destructive forces are mutually dependent. Everything in the external environment has some impact on how the body ages internally. And the body's diminished ability to cope with injury affects its vulnerability to external injury.

In fact, in 1993 I was one of the first people to talk about "environmental aging." By that term I meant aging that results from the combination of external injury and compromised internal cellular functions. I believe we have the ability to slow environmental aging, and that sun protection on the outside of our skin isn't our only weapon.

Of course, protecting the skin from the most serious environmental insult—overexposure to sunlight—can begin immediately with proper use of sunscreen. But the skin's defenses can also be boosted internally, by taking an antioxidant supplement, such as pomegranate extract. In chapter 9, you will learn how ellagic acid, one of the key active ingredients in pomegranate extract, works internally to increase the sun protection factor (SPF) of your topical sunscreen by 25 percent.

REJUVENATION

The core component of the program is improving your skin's internal environment so that it can function at its very best. As a result, the visible signs of aging will fade, but the main purpose is to give your skin a healthy environment so that it can heal itself. This program is not based on a single component but on a combination of anti-aging steps:

- It hydrates skin cells with water-attracting and water-holding molecules.
- It disarms free radicals with specific antioxidants before they can damage skin structures.
- It reduces inflammation with skin soothers, which also curtail free radical production.

- It repairs damage to connective tissue with amino acids, minerals, vitamins, and other nutrients.
- It provides key nutrients, such as fatty acids, to repair damaged cell membranes and prevent water loss.

Some of the nutrients and botanicals you'll be learning about are taken internally every day. Some are applied to your skin's surface at least twice a day. And some require weekly or monthly treatments.

STAYING ON THE PROGRAM

Patients and Murad Spa clients tell me that the program quickly becomes part of the everyday routine. The hardest steps, I'm told, are taking time out to relax every day and the weekly facial treatment. We seem to be a nation of doers, and doing nothing for just fifteen minutes while the vitamin C infusion seeps in, or practicing deep breathing exercises, is very difficult. When people tell me this step is so difficult, it tells me a great deal about why their skin appears dull, old, and etched with worry lines. People who can't stop for fifteen minutes a week to care for themselves are under enormous stress. And from what I'm told by my patients, many of you are in this situation.

What you are going to learn how to do in the pages that follow is to accomplish six anti-aging skin care objectives:

- increasing the water content of the skin cells and hydrating the top layer of dead skin cells
- increasing the rate of skin cell turnover
- flooding the skin inside and out with nutrients that counter free radical damage and inflammation
- providing the skin inside and out with the building materials needed to repair and maintain collagen and elastin fibers

- bolstering the cell membranes with fatty acids, lecithin, phosphatidylcholine, and choline
- protecting the skin inside and out from ultraviolet radiation, the major aging accelerator, and pollution

---

A SAMPLE PROGRAM

Sarah, a forty-six-year-old department store executive, came to me because she was considering a face-lift. She had recently started a new job and couldn't take the time off that's needed for a complete recovery for at least two years. Sarah was adamant about not letting anyone know she'd had surgery, and so wanted to postpone the operation until she could take "a trip to Europe." At least that was the alibi she planned to use.

Sarah wanted to know what I could do to soften her wrinkles, firm her neckline, and fade the dark blotches along her jawline. She wanted to look as good as she could until she could have a face-lift.

Sarah's skin was typical of many women who have not yet gone through menopause. Although her cheeks were a little dry, the skin was supple and moist along her forehead and down the center of her nose and chin. Occasionally, just before her period, she would get a pimple or two, but she had never been troubled with acne. She had been a serious sun worshiper until a tiny skin cancer alerted her to the dangers of tanning.

Sarah was so determined to look her best that she

followed the program for normal/combination skin religiously. She even gave herself the weekly vitamin C infusion treatment.

Sarah has been on the program for over a year, and she hasn't made a final decision about the face-lift, but she's wavering. "Now I really am considering taking a trip to Europe. Taking a month off to enjoy Italy will be healthier for me than having surgery. Besides, now that my blotches are gone and I don't have so many lines around my eyes, I think I can postpone a face-lift for a couple more years."

TWO

Skin 101

You were born with robust skin cells that divide regularly and adhere neatly to one another, covering your body. But the skin is not just a protective envelope. It's a functioning organ, and like your lungs, liver, and brain, it has chores to do. It regulates your body temperature. It communicates sensations, allowing you to feel a cool breeze and pull back from a hot stove before you get burned.

Skin is also an important defender. It makes pigment to shield its fragile genetic material from radiation. Some of its cells are like soldiers, guarding against invaders and, when necessary, signaling other cells to release defensive proteins and alerting the body's immune system. You'll learn more about this inflammatory response later, because it also contributes to the changes in skin that we call "aging."

While skin is doing its many jobs, it's also sustaining itself. Sebaceous glands secrete sebum to keep it lubricated, and an internal hydration system keeps the moisture level in balance. Skin is also constantly repairing and renewing itself so that it doesn't wear out or break down. It circulates natural antioxidants to squelch free radicals, and it breaks down nutrients to essential molecules that give each cell precisely what it needs.

Skin is your largest organ, comprising about 16 percent of your total body weight. Every square inch of skin on your face contains about 65 hairs, 100 oil glands, 650 sweat glands, 78 yards of nerves, and 19 yards of blood vessels.

I've mentioned earlier that the skin is a kind of factory. Just as an automobile plant uses raw materials such as steel, rubber, and plastic to make a car, so the skin needs a steady supply of sugar, water, and proteins to make cells and the materials that hold them together.

In order for a factory to turn out goods, it needs machinery and the electricity and oil to keep the equipment working. Your skin needs fuel also. It has fats and amino acids to maintain its metabolism, and B vitamins and trace minerals, among other things, to maintain its structures. It also needs antioxidants to prevent those structures from a kind of biological rusting.

I believe that to keep this factory running efficiently and maintaining its physical structures, it must be constantly supplied with raw materials. And, because the factory becomes more inefficient with age, you need to increase its supply of raw materials as time goes by.

FRESH AS A BABY'S CHEEKS, AND THEN . . . .

Unlike your other organs, skin is visible. Or at least its surface is. You can tell at a glance from its color and texture whether it's healthy and vital. You can also make a good guess at how old it is.

We all begin life with the same structural and cellular equipment. The moist, smooth skin covering the rosy, plump cheeks of a young baby is nearly irresistible. We want to reach out and feel that lovely surface. Although adolescent breakouts may mar it later, the skin functions and appears healthy and robust until about age twenty-five. But from that point until about the sixth decade, the skin goes through a remarkable decline.

The skin of an elderly person has thinned and stretched, while the supporting fatty cushion, bones, and other tissues beneath it have gradually shrunken. Like wallpaper that's too big for the space it is to cover, the skin drapes and bunches in all the wrong places. As skin separates from underlying muscle and tissue on the face, it hangs loosely from the forehead, the cheekbones, and the jawline. The color is dull, maybe even yellowish. Dark spots and blotches disrupt the surface, indicating that some of the pigment-producing cells have worn out, and others are trying to compensate for the loss. Sadly, this is not skin you want to touch.

But not every older person's skin appears this way. Think of someone who is older but whose skin is still lovely. Perhaps some fat has been lost, and there are some loose folds, but the skin tone is even and the complexion is bright. There are several reasons for the differences you see among older people.

It's partly in the genes. The genes you inherited from your parents have an enormous impact on the rate at which you will age and how all of your organs, including your skin, will perform. Even your reaction to environmental factors is partly a reflection of your genetic makeup.

Think about your father, your grandmother, and your older sister. Does your grandmother have lovely smooth skin or is she covered with age spots and deep wrinkles? How did your parents and grandparents' skin react to sunlight? If they protected themselves, is their skin still smooth and their complexion bright? If they didn't, and they spent a lot of time outdoors, do they have thick, deeply wrinkled skin, or is their complexion fairly free of wrinkles and blotches? Is there skin cancer in your family? As you recall your family's histories and look at old photographs, you'll catch glimpses of yourself that predict many of your own visible signs of aging—those you want to start preventing right now.

While giving genetics its due, I believe that the most important influence on how your skin ages is how well you care for it—inside and out. Your genetic heritage may be your starting point, but you can modify the risks your inherited genes have placed on you. For example, a person with a family history of heart disease has a good chance of overcoming their risk and reducing their chances of having a heart attack by keeping a healthy weight, lowering the level of the harmful type of cholesterol in the blood, eating healthy, fiber-rich foods, and exercising regularly. You can do the same for your skin.

SKIN-DEEP

To understand the hows and whys of good skin care, it's useful to know some basics about how skin cells are made and what skin looks like on a microscopic level. Also, as you learn more about my program, you'll be hearing how the steps I'm going to recommend affect specific layers of the skin to help renew, rejuvenate, and protect it. You'll also understand why my approach is both internal and external.

In the illustration that follows, you can see that the skin is made of several layers and that each layer has several sub-layers. At the very bottom is an insulating cushion of fat.

Next, and making up about 90 percent of the skin, is the dermis. It contains most of the supportive collagen and stretchy elastin that give skin its structure. Here, too, are fibroblasts that churn out more collagen and elastin to replenish these fibers. The dermis is about 60 percent water and a gel-like mix of various nourishing and moisture-holding molecules.

Above the dermis is the epidermis. Skin cells at the bottom, or *basal*, layer of the epidermis divide, and over the next month or so new daughter cells move up, pushing an old cell up ahead of

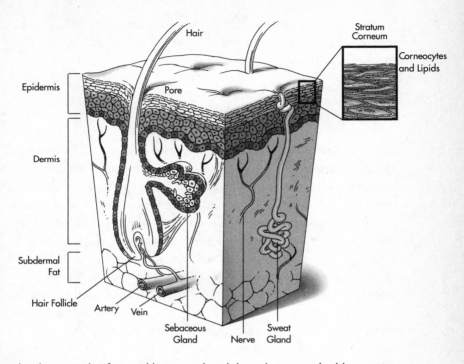

The skin is made of several layers and each layer has several sublayers. At the very bottom is an insulating cushion of fat.

it. As the new cells move upward through the epidermis, they mature and develop more protein, or keratin, as they go. Some of the lipids, or fats, within the cell are released into the space between the cells, which helps the cells stay plump and moist. Then, near the top, these cells, now called *keratinocytes,* will begin to die. At the very top, there are about twenty-five layers of dead skin cells. This is the part of the epidermis that you see. It's called the *stratum corneum.* Eventually, the dead cells are sloughed off and replaced by new ones.

You have probably heard this eight-week process described as "cell turnover." It takes place in the epidermis continuously, but the rate at which it occurs gradually slows by 30 to 50 percent by the time you're eighty years old.

THE ULTIMATE BARRIER

Over my thirty years of practicing dermatology, I have come to realize that everything I do to help people renew, rejuvenate, and protect their skin is based on two basic principles: to maintain the barrier function of the skin and to help the skin hold as much water as possible. I'm going to return to this concept repeatedly throughout this book, so you don't have to be concerned with remembering it. For now, though, as you read about how skin ages, you'll see how the events that occur within the skin layers over time affect the skin's barrier function and its ability to hold water.

The Top Layer. Throughout life, the constantly turning over layer of dead skin cells that rests on top of the epidermis, the stratum corneum, doesn't change much. Studies have shown that this layer may thin slightly with age, but it remains protective and, if well cared for, will adequately prevent moisture loss from the layers beneath it. Dead cells do tend to linger longer on the surface of skin as you age, which is why older skin feels rougher than young skin.

Pigment Production. Earlier I explained that skin contains pigment to protect it from the sun. The cells that produce this pigment, known as melanin, are called *melanocytes,* and they make up about 3 percent of the cells in the epidermis. Each melanocyte provides melanin for about thirty-six skin cells. The number of active melanocytes decreases by an estimated 10 to 20 percent per decade of adult life. The melanocytes that remain attempt to compensate for the missing ones, so you have an overproduction of pigment in one area and a decline or complete absence of melanin in another. This is why age spots form and skin becomes splotched with darker and lighter shades of color.

Infection Fighters. The number of *Langerhans' cells* also decreases. These cells in the epidermis are major players in the skin's immune response. It's their job to spot foreign substances or microorganisms and mark them for attack. According to some estimates, as much as half of the skin's supply of Langerhans' cells are lost by late adulthood, which may explain why older skin is more susceptible to infection and skin cancer.

Skin Anchors. There are age-related changes, where the epidermis meets the dermis. Tiny projections of tissue from the dermis into the epidermis hold the two together like the joints in the leaves of a table. Over time, these projections flatten. The two skin layers no longer share nutrients and moisture-holding molecules as easily as they once did. Also, the two layers aren't as tightly attached as they were when the skin was younger; a minor injury can separate them. That is why older people's skin blisters more easily than young skin.

Blood Vessels. With aging, the blood vessels that carry nutrients and moisture to the skin diminish and their structure changes. Sun damage makes the change in blood vessels even worse. For example, experiments have shown that sunlight causes blood vessel walls to thicken. Eventually, as they dilate, you can see them. They look like tiny red threads just under the skin's surface.

Moisture-Holding Molecules. The matrix of protein fibers (see "Collagen and Elastin" below) in the dermis is embedded in a gel-like material called *ground substance.* If the dermis were a mud roof, the fibers of collagen and elastin would be the straw, and the ground substance the mud that holds it all together. In this "mud" are various moisture-holding molecules of complex sugars and protein called *glycosaminoglycans* (GAGs). The different water-loving molecules that make up GAGs keep everything they surround moist, and that moisture is essential to skin functioning. For instance, moisture in the dermis and epidermis keeps the collagen and elastin pliable. Over time, there's a slight natural decrease in the amount of ground substance in the skin, and even more is lost when there is excessive sun exposure.

Collagen and Elastin. Most of the signs of aging you see begin in the tough, fibrous dermis. The meshwork is largely bundles of thin, white collagen fibers interspersed with wavy, branching, rubbery fibers of elastin. Collagen and elastin form the skin's infrastructure and give it strength and resiliency. With aging, though, the number of fibroblasts that make collagen and elastin decrease, and skin repair slows down. Fibroblasts are also affected by the decline in ground substance, which is their source of building materials such as amino acids.

In fact, it was aging researcher Leonard Hayflick's experiments with fibroblasts from the skin of fetuses in the early 1960s that led to one of the widely accepted theories of why we age. Hayflick discovered that our cells divide a predictable and finite number of times. When they stop, we age.

The main building materials of the dermis—the collagen, elastin, and ground substance—are found in other parts of the body as well, such as in the connective tissue of ligaments and tendons. Later, when you learn about how to boost the health of the skin with internal skin care, you also will see how other parts of the body benefit as well.

INVISIBLE DAMAGE

Wrinkles begin forming years before they are etched in the skin or the force of gravity becomes obvious. Some of the cellular changes are part of the inevitable slowdown that occurs throughout the body, but in the skin, there is another factor that speeds the aging process. It's the inflammation caused by sunlight and harsh treatment. The damage created by inflammation will be described in more detail later, but for now let's look at what happens to collagen and elastin in response to age and sunlight. That's where much of the action is for wrinkles.

Elastin. According to some experts, the earliest and most profound aging changes occur in the elastin fibers. As we grow older, the strong, hollow fibers take on what is often described as a "moth-eaten" appearance. The fibers also gradually thicken and curl. Normally, elastin fibers reach out to each other with delicate branches. With age, however, the branches become tough and disorderly and finally degenerate into a tangled mass.

As the fine elastic fibers become rigid and thick, the skin loses its elasticity. The elastin fibers become like a bunch of rubber bands that have become dried out and old at the bottom of your desk drawer. There is still the same number, but they don't stretch as far or snap back as quickly, and they break apart easily. These changes in elastin occur in everyone, but in skin that is exposed to ultraviolet radiation from the sun, the elastin is very distorted.

Although overall, the skin thins with age, the structure of elastin changes and can actually cause skin to thicken in some areas, especially those exposed to too much sun. This is called *solar elastosis*.

In one study elastin fibers from the sun-protected skin of the buttocks were compared to those of young skin. In sun-exposed skin from the forearm, the elastin fibers were twenty times thicker than normal.

By middle age, most Caucasians have severe elastin degeneration. Sun exposure creates those changes even earlier. Skin biopsies from young people who spend a lot of time in the sun show that advanced degeneration can occur by the early twenties. These changes are sometimes called "invisible damage," because the tangled masses of protein fibers won't cause a noticeable change for many years.

Collagen. While elastin fibers are becoming more distorted and tangled, collagen is decreasing at the rate of about 1 percent per year. Strong collagen fibers are in tendons and ligaments, but in skin, the fibers also provide a degree of thickness. Because women have less collagen than men do, their skin is about fifteen years older, from a structural point of view, than men's skin.

With age, collagen becomes even thicker, especially if there has been significant sun exposure. In young skin, single fibers of collagen are organized into bundles. With age, the bundles of collagen fibers become larger and are stacked every which way. The fine meshwork that characterizes young collagen becomes ropy and misshapen. The fibers stretch out of shape like overused old rubber bands.

Chewing Up Protein. Ironically, the chaos of thick and tangled collagen and elastin deep within the skin is turned on by a rather orderly aging process. Certain genes switch on the production of enzyme-secreting cells in the dermis. These enzymes literally chew up collagen and elastin. Later, when we discuss how vitamins applied to the skin and taken internally can improve fine lines and wrinkles, you'll understand why being able to subdue these enzymes is so important.

Several things activate these enzymes. One is the inflamma-

SMOKING AND YOUR SKIN

A kind of damage similar to aging occurs in people who smoke. Studies have shown that heavy smokers are nearly five times more likely to be wrinkled than nonsmokers are. Part of the reason is those notorious collagen-destroying enzymes. Skin cells in a test tube that was exposed to a smoke-saturated salt water made more of the enzymes than normal, and the fibroblasts were 40 percent less efficient than normal in producing new collagen.

But that's not all smoking does to skin. So-called cigarette skin is pale, thick, and has a grayish hue with wrinkles and folds most noticeable on the cheeks. One reason for this is that nicotine causes the blood vessels to contract, so less oxygen-bearing blood reaches the skin. Smoking also increases production of elastin by about 100 percent, but the new elastin is thicker than normal. Finally, smoking repeatedly contracts the skin as the person purses their lips, tightens their facial muscles, and squints to avoid the irritating smoke. Bending the collagen repeatedly in this way creates permanent bends and breaks, or smoker's wrinkles.

---

tion of sunburn. A study done at the University of Michigan a few years ago showed that a single dose of ultraviolet light, equivalent to five to fifteen minutes of exposure to the noonday sun, dramatically increased the level of these collagen-destroying enzymes in the skin within eight hours. It took nearly seventy-two hours after the blast of sunlight for the level of enzymes to return to normal. When the skin was bombarded with UV radiation every two days for several sessions, the enzyme levels remained unusually high for a week. Just think what a summer of suntanning does to the collagen in your skin.

Aging also causes an increase in these enzymes. Here's how it works: As skin cells age, they no longer produce enough genetic material (DNA) to allow the cells to divide as quickly and completely as they once did. By the time you're seventy or eighty, you have clusters of these sluggish old cells deep within the skin. At twenty-five or thirty, you probably had none.

These worn-out old cells don't just hang around taking up space. They are destructive because they churn out collagen-chewing enzymes. One reason wrinkles form is that collagen and elastin are being destroyed, and repair of the fibers has slowed. Remember that those collagen and elastin factories—the fibroblasts—are diminishing, too.

THE BIG PICTURE OF AGING SKIN

The aging signs you see in the mirror are a reflection of events taking place on a microscopic level. It's important to understand this concept, because what you're going to do to reverse and repair your aging skin will take place first in the cells of these layers and will take at least five weeks to become noticeable.

Here are just a few of the changes that typically begin at about age twenty to twenty-five:

- The individual skin cells that are being made are larger and their shape is more irregular. They also develop more slowly.
- There are fewer layers of dead cells on the surface.

- There is a decrease in the water-holding molecules sur-rounding the collagen and elastin that keeps them pliable and moist.
- There is a decrease in the water-holding molecules that surround the developing skin cells and the dead cells of the skin's top layer.
- The pigment-producing cells become 20 percent less dense every ten years. At the same time there is an increase in melanin production in small areas, which is the cause of age spots.
- The immune cells of the skin that help protect it, the Langer-hans' cells, diminish by half between young adulthood and old age, and they are further diminished by sun exposure.
- The cells called fibroblasts that produce collagen and elastin become less active.
- The collagen fibers that give skin its resiliency become thicker and more brittle and decrease by about 1 percent a year.
- Elastin fibers that give skin its elasticity become loose and break easily. There are also fewer of them.
- The ground substance that holds the collagen and elastin fibers together thins.
- Blood vessels that carry nutrients and remove cellular waste from the skin diminish. Those that remain may become dilated and their walls may thicken. They tend to twist and break.

SKIN SELF-EXAM

The big picture is the visible age-related changes in your skin that trouble you. What do you see when you look at your face in the mirror? What would you like to improve?

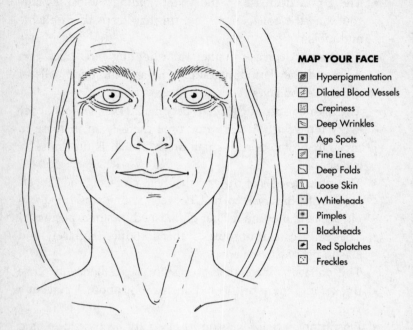

MAP YOUR FACE

- Hyperpigmentation
- Dilated Blood Vessels
- Crepiness
- Deep Wrinkles
- Age Spots
- Fine Lines
- Deep Folds
- Loose Skin
- Whiteheads
- Pimples
- Blackheads
- Red Splotches
- Freckles

Use this face map of aging signs to guide you in mapping your face on page 36.

- Do you have rough, dry areas on your skin?
- Do you have areas that seem thicker? Thinner?
- Do you have growths or moles?
- Are some areas of your face darker or lighter than others?
- Can you see fine lines around your eyes? Above your upper lip? Along your cheeks?
- Do you have tiny goose bumps on your neck? Does it appear crepey?

- Can you see tiny, threadlike blood vessels on your cheeks or at the sides of your nose?
- Do you have deep lines running from the corners of your nose to the corners of your mouth? From the corners of your mouth down either side of your chin? Between your eyebrows? Across your forehead?

Now look at the rest of your body.

- Do you have rough, dry skin on your elbows, knees, and feet?
- Do you bruise or bleed easily?
- Pinch the skin on your hand. Does it take more than a second to return to its normal position?
- Do you have dry, brittle nails?
- Is the skin on your legs rough and scaly?

Each of these questions touches on a visible sign of aging. To mark your progress as you follow the program, use the face map to document your starting point.

Wash your face, but don't put on any moisturizer or makeup. An hour later, pull back your hair, turn on the lights, and examine every square inch of your face. Look straight ahead, and then take a hand mirror to see the sides of your face from the top of your hairline down to your neck.

Unlike weight loss or exercise, the progress you make by following a skin care plan can't be easily measured. Before-and-after pictures help, but for now the only objective measures in the texture of your skin, in the depths of your wrinkles, are costly ones in the laboratories where skin care products are developed. You are the best judge of the improvements seen and felt in your skin, so keeping this visual diary will help you mark your progress.

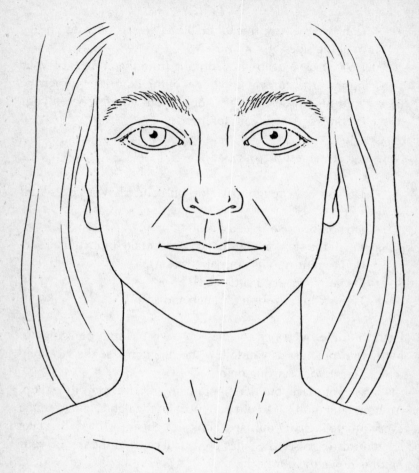

When you look in the mirror again in five weeks, you're going to notice that many of these visible signs of aging have improved. In another five weeks, you'll notice even more improvement. But also make a note somewhere about how your skin feels. Does your makeup go on more smoothly? Do you find yourself going without makeup more often because your skin has a new brightness? These subjective improvements are as important to recognize as the changes you see in the mirror.

WHY SKIN AGES

We're fortunate to live at a time when nearly a century of research is beginning to unravel the mysteries of aging. For instance, it's now known that some key steps are built in to the machinery of each cell of our body. From an evolutionary point of view, it's as if we're programmed to self-destruct after our reproductive years have passed. By the time we reach seventy-five, we have about 30 percent fewer cells than we started with.

From the point of view of evolution, our purpose on earth is to produce offspring and to stay around long enough to raise them so that they can reproduce and thus carry on our genetic heritage. So, with evolution in mind, it makes sense that we look our best and are most attractive to the opposite sex when we are in our early reproductive years, say late teens to mid-twenties. We then begin to age as our ability to reproduce reaches a peak.

About three hundred theories of aging have been suggested, of which at least a dozen explain why cells decline. The most likely theory is that cells lose their ability to reproduce because of accumulated damage. That damage is caused by several forces, with destructive rogue molecules called free radicals at the top of the list.

Another leading theory is that cells become less able to digest their own waste products, and the odd bits and pieces of cellular sludge gum up the works. The accumulated debris is called *lipofuscin*.

The newest theory is that the tips (or *telomeres*) of the cell's forty-six chromosomes—the long strings of genes in the center of the cell—get shorter and shorter each time the chromosomes are duplicated as the cell divides. Eventually the shortened chromosome is destabilized and may break apart. Some scientists believe that the telomere on the chromosome tip is the clock that keeps track of cell division. And, as Hayflick discovered, the number of cell divisions is limited.

Most likely all three theories—and probably more—are true. But the net effect of all of them is water loss. Water is lost from within the cells. Water is lost from the material that keeps the collagen and elastin factories going. Water is lost from every layer of the skin.

I believe that an inclusive program counters all the causes of this water loss. Free radicals that damage the cell membranes, allowing water to seep out, can be disarmed. Anti-inflammatory agents can reduce the formation of free radicals created by inflammation. Hydrating agents can help supply the skin with water-attracting and water-holding molecules while protecting the cell membrane and connective tissue. And nutrients can help prevent water loss: lecithin replenishes cell membranes, and glucosamine and amino acids maintain connective tissues.

Of course, free radicals are important. In fact, free radicals are implicated in nearly every breakdown that occurs in the human body, and they directly damage various structures within the skin.

Molecules on the Loose. Free radicals are unstable molecules or parts of molecules within cells. There is still no evidence in human studies that getting rid of free radicals before they cause too much damage will actually extend life, but many experiments have shown that curtailing their unruly behavior can slow age-related changes.

Free radicals are powerful destroyers because they break up other molecules, which creates even more free radicals. A molecule consists of bundles of atoms that have a certain number of electrons in their outer shells. They're in balance and humming along, performing their tasks. But in doing some of those jobs, the molecules lose electrons. To restore their balance, they bombard other molecules in hopes of stealing the much-needed electron.

So while one free radical manages to rebalance or neutralize itself, other destructive free radicals are created. The damage accumulates and the cells begin to malfunction and age.

Any molecule can become a free radical, but the most common is oxygen. That's right, the same life-giving molecule that is so essential to our well-being can also become a toxic destroyer. Oxygen free radicals are constantly being formed, and they search incessantly for an accessible electron that will restore their stability.

Free radicals can destroy protein, fats in the cell walls, and DNA at the cell's core. Virtually any part of the cell is easy prey, but most susceptible are polyunsaturated fatty acids. Disturbing this important component of the cell ultimately affects the cell's integrity.

Free radicals are created within the cell in many ways. Some are the unavoidable side effect of the cell's own metabolism. But free radicals are also created by other reactions, such as inflammation. Anything that increases the use of oxygen, like strenuous exercise, or creates a molecular disturbance in the cell, such as pollution, cigarette smoke, heat, radiation, and ultraviolet light, forms free radicals. So does alcohol, eating too much iron, and high-fat diets.

Luckily, nature has also provided us with a defense system for keeping free radicals in check. There are enzymes circulating in the body that can prevent the formation of free radicals or force free radicals to join forces and give balance to each other. In addition, there are molecules that carry extra electrons to give to free radicals when necessary. These generous, electron-sharing molecules are called antioxidants.

Preventing free radicals from forming and neutralizing or disarming those that do occur is an essential part of my anti-aging skin care program. And, as you'll be learning as you follow each step of the program, I believe there are two ways of stopping free radical damage. One is to prevent free radicals from forming in the first place by protecting the body from the assaults that create them, such as inflammation. The second anti-aging step is to flood the skin with antioxidants internally and externally to disarm as many freewheeling, free radical molecules as possible.

Unlike skin care programs that rely only on surface treatments, this program benefits the entire body. Because as you consume supplements and fruits and vegetables to saturate the skin with antioxidants from the inside, you are also targeting free radicals in the blood vessels, brain, lungs, and other organs.

Fighting free radicals and inflammation and stimulating collagen production are the cutting edge of anti-aging skin care today. We know from countless studies in animals and humans that significant improvements can make your skin look years younger and slow the rate of aging. But there is still no fountain of youth that will extend life. At best, we know that people can live as long as 122 years. My goal, and that of other skin care and aging researchers, is to keep you healthy and looking youthful for as long as possible. As anthropologist Ashley Montagu said, "The goal in life is to die young as late as possible."

THREE

The Water Principle

Throughout this book, the main purpose underlying everything I suggest you do for your skin is to make it—and your body—healthier. Healthy skin is clear, luminous, and beautiful. Once you achieve that goal, there's another challenge: keeping your skin defenses strong.

Your skin is your body's protective envelope, and it is constantly under attack inside and out. On the outside, toxic chemicals and pollution, ultraviolet radiation in sunlight, agents that cause inflammation, and free radicals in the atmosphere bombard the skin's surface. Inside, natural enzymatic reactions, inflammatory responses, and free radicals formed within the skin do their damage.

Your job—day and night, inside and out—is continual repair and maintenance. Though keeping up with skin's demands may sound like drudgery, it isn't. It can be accomplished in just five minutes or less, twice a day. Once you get your personal routine down, you'll do it as automatically as you brush your teeth. Skin care—and improving the health of your body while you're at it—

doesn't have to become an obsession. You can quickly do each step of the program in the morning and again at night, and then forget about it. Until, of course, a friend says about a month from now, "You look different. Have you had something done?"

In my practice, at my spa, and in the products I've developed, my primary concern is helping people maintain the barrier function of their skin and keeping the cells supplied with water. I believe that water is the most important factor in an anti-aging program. As a result of my research and practice caring for thousands of men, women, and children with every skin condition imaginable, I have developed the following recipe for keeping skin cells hydrated. Your daily program should consist of:

- antioxidants to disarm free radicals, which ultimately damage the cell membrane and cause it to lose water
- anti-inflammatory agents to reduce inflammation, which releases free radicals that damage cellular structures and cause water loss
- natural moisture factors to absorb water from the environment and act as a reservoir for water in the skin
- hydrophobic agents such as ceramides, which prevent water loss from all cells and maintain the skin's barrier function—these can also be essential in repairing and maintaining cell membranes
- fatty acid and glucosamine supplements to encourage the body to make its own water-holding molecules
- lecithin, and its building blocks phosphatidylcholine and choline to maintain cell walls

Having all of these ingredients in an internal and external skin care program will help maintain the water balance in your entire body.

If you're eager to get started, you can jump ahead and find

the regimen and the recommendations that suit you in chapter 12. But later or right now, I think it's helpful for you to understand the basic principle underlying my program. I call it *The Water Principle*. Once you get it, your entire approach to caring for yourself will change.

SKIN IS A WATER GAUGE

The Water Principle is not about drinking four or eight or twelve glasses a day, though I will share my thoughts about drinking water with you in a moment. I'm talking about getting water into cells and keeping it there so that every one of the trillions of cells in your body functions at full capacity.

Next to oxygen, water is the most important substance you need, and almost everything we know about aging tells us that the decline in function over the years is a story of water loss. At birth, about 75 percent of our weight is water, but gradually as we age we lose the ability to hold on to water. On average, man is about 60 percent water. A 15 percent decrease in water may not seem like much, but as you'll see, if we look at the cheeks of a baby and a seventy-year-old, it makes a dramatic, visible difference.

The skin is the largest and only visible organ of the body, and it reflects the aging processes—including water loss—that occur throughout the body. When I see dry, thin, sagging skin, I know that the problem doesn't stop there. The damaged, water-deprived fibers and cells, and the gel-like substance in which they are all embedded, tell me that a similar situation exists in the cells of the heart, the muscles, the liver, the walls of the blood vessels, and the joints. Each and every cell of the body is connected. Therefore, if water is lost from the epidermis, those cells will withdraw water from somewhere else. It comes from the fluid circulating around the cells, then from an adjacent cell or from the dermis beneath it, and eventually from other tissues or cells of other organs.

When I was in medical school, I learned that one of the quickest ways to tell if a patient was dehydrated was to gently pinch the skin on the back of the hand, lift it up, and then let go. If it failed to rebound instantly, the person needed more fluids. This test worked well in most young adults, but in older people, the skin reacted as if they were dehydrated even when I knew they weren't. That little pinch of skin formed a peak on their hands that lasted a full second, perhaps even longer if the person's skin was very sun-damaged. Their skin cells had long ago lost the ability to hold on to water, and structures that gave skin its resiliency had suffered irreparable harm as a result.

I learned in my years caring for very sick patients that while the body may have a survivor mechanism that keeps water in the cells of the most vital organs, if there is a lack of water in the skin, chances are there's a shortage elsewhere in the body as well.

Water is essential to the life of every living cell. It is what keeps a cell from collapsing in on itself, so one of the purposes of the body's natural chemistry is to insure that each cell from the brain to the heart to the organs of the abdomen are kept plump with fluid on the inside and lubricated with moisture on the outside. Water also gives volume to the blood and pliability to the tissues. You can see this in your skin.

Without an adequate water supply, the skin cells disintegrate. Structures that support skin become stiff and lose flexibility. The skin layers become thin and flat. Blood vessel walls become fragile, porous, and leak water like old pipes. Nutrients can't be delivered, and waste materials aren't carried away. And the more water that's lost, the more fragile and penetrable the barrier is. That weakening means even more water is lost, and a destructive, self-perpetuating cycle is set in motion.

You can put a stop to this water loss. You can rebuild a vital strong barrier that not only gives you a more youthful appearance but also functions at its full potential, defending itself against further water loss.

THE MISSING LINK

In recent years you've probably heard a lot about free radicals and inflammation. Millions of dollars and the most brilliant minds in the world have been unraveling the mystery of how these forces cause your body—and your skin—to self-destruct. And not only are inflammation and free radicals inextricably linked to wrinkles and the aging process in general, they are important players in chronic diseases from diabetes to arthritis to cancer. But as important as these factors are, there is much more to health—or to be more precise, the loss of health and degeneration of the body—than just inflammation or free radical damage.

In the human body a problem in one area leads to a problem in another; one missing link, one injury or deficiency, makes an impact on another vital function. Scientists are likely to find that along with free radicals and inflammation, which we know we can do something about right now, there are other forces at work. There may be many causes, but I believe they all culminate in one disastrous result: water loss. In my mind it is the missing link in understanding how aging affects health and beauty.

Whether I talk about the destruction of the skin's surface layer by free radicals in the environment, the inflammation triggered deep within the skin by sunburn, or the thinning and weakening of the blood vessels that supply the skin, the net effect of them all is a loss of water. You can see this happening in your own skin, because it leads to wrinkles, flakiness, fine lines, discoloration, puffiness, and laxity.

I believe that all cells have a commonality. A liver cell, a heart cell, and a skin cell have different purposes but they share one thing in common—they are containers filled with *cytoplasm,* which is mostly water. All the cells of the body need their full complement of water to function at their optimum capacity. If one organ or system is deficient in this water, it will take the water from other tissues.

You will be learning in the following chapters about free radicals and inflammation and how they play an important role in aging skin, mostly because they damage the membranes of the cell wall. When these membranes are damaged, the water in the cytoplasm begins to seep out. The cell, then, is less efficient and more susceptible to disease.

ABOUT THAT EIGHT GLASSES

If you're a woman, about 50 percent of your body weight is water. If you're a man, it's 60 percent. And most of that water (about 40 percent of it) is within your body's cells. Obviously, of all the raw materials you need, water is at the top of the list of the forty-odd other ones. To keep that healthy water level available to all your cells, common wisdom is that you should drink a couple of quarts of replenishing water a day. That's where the adage to

drink eight glasses of water a day comes from. But I've found little scientific evidence for this advice. In fact, in 2002 a Dartmouth
Medical School professor and kidney specialist reported in the
American Journal of Physiology that after reviewing the scientific
literature he found no evidence to support the commonly known
"eight by eight" rule that advises drinking eight eight-ounce
glasses of water a day. In fact, the published studies suggest that
large amounts of water are not needed. What is known for certain
is that it's extremely difficult to drink too much water. If you
manage to swallow more than ten glasses of water one after
another very quickly, you might end up with a condition called
water intoxication, but that is pretty hard to do.

The more water you drink, you've no doubt noticed, the more
trips you make to the bathroom to get rid of the excess. Healthy
kidneys are miracles of filtration, and these two, fist-size organs
are designed to insure that your water reservoir stays full but not
overfull. If you run a 5K race and lose a lot of water in sweat, the
kidneys let more water flow back into your system. If you sip on
tea and soda all day, the excess water gets filtered out. If you're
drinking large amounts of water to keep that full feeling in your
stomach, as many diet programs recommend, you're going to
make more trips to the bathroom than to the refrigerator. It's
annoying, but it can't hurt you.

However, every time your kidneys or sweat glands work, you
lose not only vital water but also other substances called elec-
trolytes. Think about spraying your face with water—as you let it
evaporate, it takes with it lipids and minerals. Every time you uri-
nate you excrete toxins, but you can also lose vital minerals.

Drinking eight glasses of water may have some health advantages. A study has shown, for instance, that men who drank more
than that had nearly half the risk of bladder cancer as those who
drank half as much. If following the eight-glasses-a-day rule
helps you to consume enough water, that's fine. However, most of

us have difficulty in drinking that much water—even four glasses may be hard—therefore, you must remember that there are other sources of water. There is water in food—especially fruits and vegetables, and eating more of them will also deliver healthful antioxidants, fiber, and other nutrients. Other beverages, like milk and juice, also contain water.

For most healthy people, the problem with water is not that we don't drink enough, it's that we may not be doing the best job of getting our cells to hold on to what we do consume. One way to insure that water stays within cells is to take fatty acids and glucosamine in a supplement. By keeping the lipid membranes surrounding the cells in good repair, the water content within that cell wall is maintained.

Many years ago while hiking, I became very thirsty and realized that even though I had been drinking a lot of water, I was perspiring and urinating more than usual. My mouth felt dry and I couldn't seem to quench my thirst. I wasn't in any danger of dehydration, but this experience made me think about how critical water is to life. We all know you can survive quite a while without food, but you won't last long without water. As I thought more and more about this, not only from the point of view of the entire organism of myself but also from the perspective of each organ, system, and cell, I realized that supplying the body with water isn't enough. I thought that holding on to water is probably one of the most rejuvenating, health-promoting things we can do. So I devised a water-holding plan that works for me.

Before a hike, I drink water and take supplements of antioxidants, glucosamine, and free fatty acids, including gamma linolenic acid, lecithin, choline, and two aspirin for the anti-inflammatory effect. (As a physician, I have worked out this regimen for myself. Before taking any nutritional supplements and aspirin, you should check with your personal physician.) This program has one major purpose: to help my cells hold on to

WATER RETENTION VERSUS HYDRATION

When I speak to people about The Water Principle, one of the first questions I'm asked, especially by women, is, "How can holding on to water be good for you?" That's because most people don't make the distinction between water inside the cells—or *intracellular* fluid—and water outside the cells—*extracellular* fluid.

Both are important for healthy skin, but excessive extracellular fluid may be unhealthy and is often unattractive. Puffy bags under the eyes, a bloated stomach, and swollen ankles are all examples of excess extracellular fluid and may signal that the body isn't handling water efficiently and that there is damage to cellular membranes. This damage can occur anywhere, such as in the blood vessels, heart, skin, liver, or muscles.

Take swollen ankles, for instance. This condition usually signals a circulatory problem. Because of a weakness in the blood vessels or heart problems or even physical pressure on the veins from sitting in one position, blood doesn't return to the heart from the legs efficiently. Instead it tends to pool in the lower extremities. Water from the blood seeps through the vein walls, as it does through old and thin rusted pipes. It accumulates in the tissues beneath the skin, causing a puffing up of the ankles and feet.

water. Nowadays when I hike with friends, they seem to need much more water than I do. I consume much less water during the hike and my mouth does not feel as dry. And I feel great afterward.

GETTING WATER INTO THE SKIN

You need to think of hydrating your skin in two ways. One, which I've just described, is to supply the deeper layers with enough water to saturate the tissues and supply the developing cells. The other is to maintain the barrier and prevent water from evaporating through the upper layers of skin and into the atmosphere.

At the very top of your skin, the dead cells stack up on top of each other like the shingles on the roof of a house, protecting the living cells of the epidermis under it, which, incidentally, is 70 percent water. Structural lipids surround these dead cells, helping to keep the cells—the shingles—in place and watertight. These structural lipids are predominately free fatty acids, ceramides, and natural moisture factors.

One way to understand the importance of your skin's barrier function is to think of your body as an apple. The skin of the apple keeps the firm flesh beneath moist and protects it from drying exposure to the air and the environment. The uppermost layer of your skin, like the peel of an apple, is a waterproof seal, keeping air out and moisture within, so the cells stay plump with fluid.

When the skin of an apple is cut or damaged, the inside of the apple begins to dry, and the exposed flesh turns brown. Even if a bump or dent so tiny that it can't be seen injures the apple skin, the flesh beneath it will become discolored.

Tiny breaks in the surface of your skin allow moisture to escape and lets in bacteria, irritants, and free radicals, all of which not only damage various structures within the skin but also accelerate further moisture loss. In the dermis, the layer of skin beneath the epidermis, are the collagen and elastin that give skin its bounce. There, too, are the fibroblasts that make these fibers. Surrounding this meshwork of fibers is a gel-like material that contains many nourishing components, and, of course, water.

Mixed in the gel are very important molecules whose job it is to pull in water. These hydrophilic or water-attracting molecules are called GAGs, an acronym for glycosaminoglycans, which you learned about in chapter 2. They are large molecules made of chains of proteins and sugars. And one of the most important of these moisture-attracting molecules is hyaluronic acid. It is found in almost all body tissues, but half of your entire body's supply is in the skin. Large quantities are also in the fluid of the joints, which is thought to diminish with age as well.

Understanding these molecules' powerful pull on water and how to increase the skin's supply of natural moisture factors, particularly GAGs, is a very active area of research for cosmetic chemists and scientists investigating the effects of aging and sun damage on skin. It's known that there are fewer of these water-attracting molecules in older skin. And we know that a loss of even a fraction of a percent means a major decline in the skin's water content because some of these molecules hold up to a thousand times their weight in water.

One way to increase the water in your skin's cells, I believe, is to supply the body with the raw materials, such as glucosamine, that it needs to manufacture water-attracting molecules like hyaluronic acid. I've discovered that in the process of increasing the amount of water in the skin, the skin is rejuvenated. Here's how it works.

If we have a sufficient amount of water in the dermis, it will be thicker and smoother. Also, cells of the other structures in your dermis—blood vessels, nerves, and glands—can function at their optimal capacity when they're well hydrated, which also encourages healthy skin. Furthermore, the dermis acts as a sponge, allowing water to be absorbed from it by the epidermis as needed. And at the same time, the dermis is a reservoir for water needed by the vital structures within it, such as sweat glands, sebaceous glands, and blood vessels.

Replenishing the water-attracting molecules in the dermis also provides nutritious soup for the fibroblasts. (You'll remember from chapter 2 that fibroblasts are the cellular factories that make collagen and elastin.) When you take the appropriate supplements (see chapter 13), you'll begin to see the result of this replenishing process in about a month, as your damaged collagen is repaired, your skin's ability to hold on to water improves, and new collagen and elastin are formed. You'll also notice a new resiliency and firmness in your skin, and the deeper wrinkles will become less obvious.

KEEPING THE BALANCE

Throughout this book, you'll be learning about ingredients that help you attract and hold water in your skin and supplements that help you boost hydration and prevent water loss. This is because I believe that water is the best antiager yet discovered. It has been established that over a lifetime our body loses a tenth of its water supply. My program is designed to help you avoid that loss and keep your skin moist and pliable. That's what young skin has going for it, and I see no reason why middle-aged and elderly skin need to suffer from dehydration.

My thirty-year career as a dermatologist has been focused on teaching people how to keep a healthy water balance in their skin—to maximize the water-holding capacity of the cells and prevent that water from escaping into the atmosphere. When I tell patients that water is money, The Water Principle becomes clear.

Think about it. If I told you that I'm going to give you ten million dollars, you'd be thrilled. But if the tax man then came and said you owed eleven million dollars in back taxes, you wouldn't be so happy. In water terms, that means you can fill your cells to their full capacity with water, but then you let it all escape, along with some of the water that was already there. Your skin—your water bank account—is in trouble, and it looks it. The same is true with your body. You can drink more water than your body can ever use, but if your cells can't save it and the water is excreted, there's no benefit in having made the effort to be well hydrated.

To keep cells healthy and hydrated, you need antioxidants, anti-inflammatory agents, collagen-builders, hydrators, and, of course, sunscreen. The products in my program incorporate this recipe. As you begin customizing your own skin care program, you'll soon see and feel how targeting each and every factor—from the external barrier of the skin (the stratum corneum) to the internal delivery of water to the dermis—affects the water content of your skin cells. You'll experience for yourself how increasing the water in your skin and your body cells rejuvenates your appearance. What you can't see, but what I think you will soon feel, is how you're also rejuvenating every cell of your body.

The external aspect of my program is designed to make the barrier of your body resilient and protective—which to the eye of the beholder is smooth, bright, and free of fine lines. That's the immediate goal, and within a day of following your new skin care regimen you're going to see visible proof of improvement. But as the next five weeks go by, you'll also see how improving the water content of your skin gives it a plumpness and clarity. You'll feel a difference in the skin's texture and elasticity.

I've always known that skin needs both internal as well as

external help to rejuvenate itself and stay healthy. And in recent years I've learned that the wrinkle-fighting steps I'm going to share with you also have a vitality-boosting impact on all your cells. And, as with the skin, the health of these cells begins and ends with water.

Wrinkle Fighters

I don't believe that basic skin care needs to be complicated, so you'll notice only minor variations between the regimens I recommend for various skin types. And you should feel free to alternate products, especially those you'll see in the "Optional" column of the regimen charts, according to your skin needs. As you will learn, an essential principle of my program is to listen to your skin. It will let you know if anything is amiss. For instance, one program may work for you during the winter but not be quite what you need in the summer, when the weather may be more humid. As long as whatever you do is gentle, doesn't damage the skin's barrier function, and is hydrating, you can't go wrong.

Keep in mind, too, that as you use my program, your skin will begin to change. It will be different in ways that you might not predict. Some of the steps or ingredients that were needed initially may not be necessary as the barrier function improves.

You have probably heard the common wisdom to "listen to your body." I think this sage advice also applies to your skin. Regardless of what you've heard, you know if your skin feels healthy and responds well to how you're treating it. Listen to your skin, and hear what it says about the products you're using. Everyone has a certain level of tolerance, a comfort zone. Know what your skin can handle. Know its limits.

SHOPPING FOR INGREDIENTS

I'll be recommending certain ingredients throughout this book. I want to caution you, though, that shopping by ingredients alone is tricky. The same ingredient in one formulation may be irritating or drying but cause no problems in a different formulation. The formulations of high-quality products are painstakingly developed so that the other ingredients counter the side effects of one ingredient. Sometimes, too, one ingredient boosts the effectiveness of another. The mix and amounts of ingredients is the *formulation,* and it can vary enormously from one product to another.

Think of a cosmetic or skin treatment product as you would a chocolate chip cookie. Yes, the chocolate chips are essential to the cookie, and the better the chocolate, the tastier the cookie will be. But if you don't also have the right mix of quality brown sugar and butter, the cookie is going to taste terrible.

Interestingly, the Rx sign that pharmacists use comes from the Latin symbol for recipe. I've developed my own recipes for skin care products for twenty years. And while individual ingredients are essential components of that formulation, it is the whole recipe that makes the product effective and safe.

In general, high-quality name brands have tested their formulations to be certain that they are safe for most skin types and that they deliver an adequate amount of the active ingredients. As with supplements, I suggest you use trusted brands of skin care products. And, finally, listen to your skin. If you react badly to a product, stop using it.

There are ingredients that accomplish each of the wrinkle-fighting steps that follow. You want the products you use as part of your daily regimen to contain as many of these rejuvenating ingredients as possible. In some products, such as cleansers, these may be in relatively low concentrations, because the objective is to cleanse your face. In other products, such as moisturizers, these ingredients are usually in higher concentrations because they are designed to leave hydrating ingredients on your skin. And some—such as antioxidants—are in very high concentrations in treatment products designed to address a specific complaint such as wrinkles, dryness, or acne.

Everything you do for your skin can deliver several of the wrinkle fighters that follow. When you wash your face, for example, you're really accomplishing two things. The obvious is that you're removing the dirt, debris, makeup, and flakes of skin cells, sweat, and sebum that have accumulated. But you can also use this cleansing step of your daily regimen to neutralize the free radicals forming in the upper layer, to begin the process of reducing inflammation, and to encourage hydration. Of course, while you're cleansing, you're also taking care not to disturb the skin's barrier function. In other words, a cleanser can do a lot more than just help rinse away oil and debris. A moisturizer can deliver more than hydrating agents. And a sunscreen can accomplish more than protecting your skin from ultraviolet radiation.

While you're taking care of your skin from the outside, you're also treating and protecting your body—and your skin—from the inside. That's why taking the supplements I suggest in chapter 13 are essential. As you read about the wrinkle fighters that follow, you'll learn how each one supports hydration inside and out.

FOUR

Hydrate

Water is so essential to our health that every organ system, including the skin, has a built-in hydrating system that is continually supplied with water from the bloodstream.

In the skin this hydrating system consists of blood vessels, sweat, and sebaceous glands, and water-holding and water-attracting molecules that work in synchrony to maintain a continuous balance between the internal water supply and the skin's demands.

As you have learned in early chapters, when the cell membranes are healthy, the cells are filled with fluid. Then each layer of skin contains hydrating molecules to keep all of its structures moist. The dermis, for instance, is kept well hydrated primarily by GAGs such as hyaluronic acid. In fact, half of the body's entire supply of water-attracting hyaluronic acid is in the dermis.

Just above the dermis is the epidermis. The skin cells divide at the base of the epidermis, and as they rise up through it, they begin to flatten and die. As they do, they slowly release their contents, the water and structural lipids inside them. So even though the superficial skin cells are no longer alive and functioning, they have structural lipids, fatty acids, cholesterol, and ceramides around them to hold on to water and keep the cells moist until they are shed. This is the outer protective shield of your body. To further assist skin hydration, water-holding sebum from the seba-ceous glands flows onto the skin's surface, creating—along with the lipids within the stratum corneum—a kind of lubricating shield that prevents water from escaping.

Skin treatment products contain some of the same hydrating molecules that are present in your skin, such as sodium pyrolli-done carboxylic acid (sodium PCA), a natural moisture factor, and ceramides.

For most healthy young people under twenty, the natural internal hydrators are sufficiently effective to keep skin plump with moisture regardless of the environmental stresses. But with aging, poor diet, and environmental damage, the skin factory becomes less and less efficient; the cellular equipment begins to break down, and the internal hydration system suffers. For instance, the hormonal shifts of age slow sebum production. GAGs, such as hyaluronic acid, diminish. And the demands of the environment may be so great that even skin that's well supplied with lipids and sebum can't keep up with the moisture loss.

Although we appreciate the appearance of moist skin, one of nature's biological purposes for keeping the cells plump with water and tightly packed is to curtail *transepidermal water loss* (TEWL). This is the loss of moisture from within the skin into the atmosphere. If that moisture can't get through the top layers of the stratum corneum, it can't escape the deeper layers of the skin. Inevitably, some of the cells' internal water supply will evaporate into the air, but if a good moisturizer and appropriate internal skin care are used consistently and adjusted according to the demands of your internal and external environment, the TEWL is kept to a minimum.

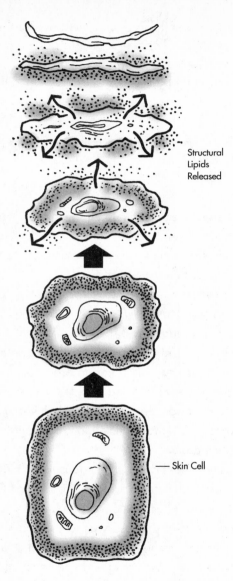

Structural
Lipids
Released

Skin Cell

As the skin cell rises up through the epidermis, it flattens and releases its contents, including water and structural lipids, into the surrounding spaces.

I believe that oily skin needs help with hydration, too. Most of the natural oil that makes skin look shiny is sebum. True, it's a natural lubricant, and since sebum is occlusive, it helps hold water in the skin, but a person with oily skin can still lack struc-

---

LIKE MOTHER, LIKE DAUGHTER

Patricia inherited her mother Janet's skin type. "Not only did I get her dry skin, I got my father's freckles," she complained when she came to see me for the eczema that had appeared on her face and hands.

"My mom had been on the Murad Program for a couple of months and I saw how much it helped her. But when I heard her best friends ask if she had a face-lift, I decided I was going to go on the program," says Patricia. Before she could start the program, I had to prescribe topical steroids and the gentlest cleansing regimen to give her skin a chance to recover from the eczema. I asked her to start taking the supplements immediately, though, and to wash her face only once a day.

Within two weeks or so, the serious inflammation was under control, and Patricia started on the Dry Skin Program, still cleansing her face only once a day.

Initially, the main purpose was to physically improve the barrier function of her skin, but long-term, I knew that Patricia needed help in coping with the stress of being a new mother. I encouraged Patricia to give herself weekly vitamin C facials and occasionally have a professional treatment at the spa. The vitamin C infusion would quickly help restore health to her skin, and the relaxation would help her eczema by subduing the stress trigger.

"The redness and peeling went away pretty quickly, and even though I don't use the medication anymore, the severe dryness hasn't come back. What really surprised me, though, was that my skin seemed to get lighter and brighter. The freckles began to fade after about a month. They haven't gone away completely, but those awful dark clusters are gone," she says.

Janet had happily encouraged Patricia to try the Murad Program because it so dramatically improved her own troubled skin.

"I never had horrible skin, but there was always something keeping it from being really nice. And as we get older, our skin doesn't get any better. But after five weeks of the vitamin C treatments people started complimenting me. 'What are you doing?' people I've known all my life would say to me. Or even more funny to me was when someone would say, 'Oh, you're one of those people who never has to worry about doing anything to your skin. It's gorgeous,' " Janet says, laughing with pride. The fine lines and wrinkles softened so much that, as Patricia said, friends starting asking if Janet had had a face-lift.

I know that Janet attributes her newly smoothed and brightened skin to the vitamin C treatments alone, but she's bolstering it twice a day with the other steps in the Dry Skin Program and with the supplements. She also uses the optional lipid serum twice a day, not just at night, which is like a superhydrator, sealing the moisture in.

tural lipids, which hydrate the deeper layers of the skin. So in certain situations—in a dry, cold, or windy climate, for instance, or when the skin is overcleansed—even skin that typically seems to have too much oil, or sebum, can become dry if not enough structural lipids are being produced.

MOISTURIZING FROM THE OUTSIDE

Keeping skin well hydrated and lubricated from the outside does several things. One, a well-formulated moisturizer can replenish the natural moisture factors in the upper layers of the skin. Two, a moisturizer helps the loose edges of the dead skin cells adhere more closely together, smoothing the skin's surface. And three, depending on the formulation, a moisturizer can leave a fine film on the skin that acts like a water-holding seal, preventing moisture from escaping into the environment. The net effect is immediately rejuvenating. It's true that the smooth, moist appearance is temporary, but if hydration is frequent and consistent, the improvements can be maintained. Of course we all would like a permanent fix, but nothing, not laser resurfacing nor a face-lift, can permanently alter the appearance, texture, and water-holding capacity of the skin. Cosmetic surgery to rejuvenate the face is basically a redraping; it doesn't affect the fabric of the skin itself. Laser and chemical peels remove surface imperfections and may increase collagen production as the skin heals, but they don't affect the skin's water-holding capacity or the size of the pores. And fillers such as fat or collagen only give the illusion of smoothness; they don't alter the way the skin performs.

Aside from looking smooth and feeling soft, hydrating the upper layers of the skin with water and moisturizing ingredients also improves the barrier function. And an intact, healthy barrier allows the skin's own moisturizing system to operate at optimum capacity. It also gives you a better defense against environmental assaults.

Imagine that the stratum corneum is the roof of your house (your body). If you keep it in good repair and the shingles (your skin cells) fit tightly next to one another, your house stays warm and dry and you stay healthy and comfortable. But if there are holes between the shingles or cracks in them, not only will your roof appear old and shabby, it will leak. Your house will be cold and damp, and heat will escape. You'll be uncomfortable and vulnerable to infections. Likewise, when there are cracks and openings in the stratum corneum, moisture escapes and free radicals and microorganisms in the environment easily penetrate. All the tiny cracks and lines in the surface become more apparent, and the dry, unprotected skin is vulnerable to injury.

SHOPPING FOR INGREDIENTS

There are roughly three thousand hydrating ingredients commonly used in over-the-counter products. Most of them aim to do what natural moisturizing factors do—that is, attract and keep water around the cells of the twenty or so layers of dead skin cells in the stratum corneum. (Although there is not a lot of water in the stratum corneum, nearly half of it is in the spaces between the cells. But the *corneocytes*, the dead skin cells, do contain a small amount of natural moisture factors.) These ingredients are called humectants. One of the most common and effective is sodium PCA, which is also found naturally in the skin.

Emollients are also hydrating. Some form a thin film on the skin's surface to hold moisture in. They also may permeate the stratum corneum and hold water there. In fact, ceramides, which make up about half of the structural lipids in the stratum corneum, can also be applied topically to increase hydration.

Glycerine is another very effective emollient. Oils such as saf-flower oil and shea butter are also helpful in holding water in the stratum corneum.

Hydrating ingredients are not limited to moisturizers. Even cleansers, which are washed away after a minute or two, can be enriched with water-holding and water-attracting ingredients that leave a moisturizing film behind. In order to gently remove the dirt and debris on your skin, some mild detergent ingredients are needed, but you don't want too much or you can take away the natural moisturizing lipids that your own skin has created. Not only do you want to avoid disturbing the skin's barrier function, you want to leave it even more hydrated than it was when you started.

Toners are another way to add hydrating ingredients to the skin along with water. A spray of a toner that contains humectant ingredients followed quickly while the skin is still damp with a hydrating moisturizer or treatment product can flood the upper layers of the skin with water and ingredients to keep it there.

Exfoliation is also helpful for moisturizing (see chapter 5), and some moisturizers contain alpha hydroxy acids to improve the health and function of the stratum corneum.

Keeping skin well hydrated is also a result of what you don't do. That means avoid products that you know irritate or dry your skin. People troubled with adult acne have a difficult time with this advice. My approach to adult acne is to first make the skin as healthy as possible by boosting its water content inside and out, then deliver acne fighters in the areas that need them; usually this is where the oil glands are most active, along the nose and chin. This is my approach to what I call *special concerns*.

The first goal is to make skin as healthy as possible so that it can efficiently work to correct and heal itself. Then, if problems persist, they can be addressed with a treatment that targets that particular problem.

HYDRATING FROM THE INSIDE

Of course you need to drink water to fuel your internal hydrating system. But beyond a certain upper limit—which differs for each person and also depends on level of activity—the excess is excreted.

While you are protecting your cells from free radicals that damage the lipids that form the cell membrane, you can also bolster that membrane with fatty acids. This is where including fish in your diet and taking omega-3 fatty acids and gamma linolenic acid supplements can help enormously. They curtail inflammation, which ultimately leads to loss of lipids from the cell membrane (see chapter 13).

Lecithin, a chemical cousin of vitamin B, is an essential building block of the lipid layer surrounding the cells and forms the foundation of the cell membrane. Lecithin is so vital to the integrity of the cell walls that the body is equipped to manufacture its own supply. We also get it from foods like soybeans, liver, cabbage, and egg yolk. In fact, the word lecithin is derived from the Greek word for egg yolk.

Phosphatidylcholine, as lecithin is sometimes called, is actually an active component of lecithin. Choline is another lecithin component.

Since liver, cabbage, and egg yolks are not on everyone's daily diet, I've added lecithin and two of its components to my hydrating supplement to help fortify the cell walls. Incidentally, there have been reports that these nutrients also improve short-term memory.

Ingredients to Look For
Sodium hyaluronate (or hyaluronic acid)
Sodium PCA

Amino acids
Plant-based lipids (phospholipids) and/or phytoceramides
Safflower seed oil
Borage seed oil
Evening primrose oil
Glycerine

Supplements
Murad Wet Suit Hydrating Supplement

FIVE

Exfoliate

Cell turnover is an ongoing process. The skin cell forms at the bottom of the epidermis, rises up through that layer, dies, and is shed. It's nudged free by wear and tear and replaced by a newly arrived cell that has completed the same process. As all of the body processes slow beginning at about age twenty, so does cell turnover. In youth the cells journey from the bottom of the epidermis to shedding, which takes about twenty-eight days. By the time you've reached late middle age, it takes about seven to ten days longer.

A week and a half doesn't seem like much, but to a dead cell hanging tenaciously to the skin's surface, it's time enough to become dried out and crinkle around the edges. That's why mature skin often feels so rough to the touch. And the irregular surface created by these flaking cells also reflects light differently, so skin appears dull and sallow, with fine lines standing out among the miniscule cracks in the surface.

Skin cells are a little like the leaves on a tree. If I pick a fresh green leaf and put water on it, the natural moisture-holding molecules in the leaf won't let anything penetrate. The water will bead up and run off, and the leaf is smooth and pliable for a while. If I put the stem in water, some of it will enter the leaf, keeping it fresh and green a little longer. Eventually, though, it will dry out.

That's what happens to the dead cells that pile up on the surface of your skin. For a while the natural moisture factors that surround them keep them supple. But eventually, exposure to the environment takes its toll. To keep that barrier strong, you have to remove those dead cells.

Exfoliation makes up for nature's slowdown by chemically or mechanically removing the topmost layer of those dead cells. To replace the shed cells, the epidermis then steps up production of new ones. The body's natural effort to keep up with this increased shedding creates healthy cells more quickly.

I believe that using an exfoliating agent to increase cell turnover to a more youthful rate is one of the best things you can do to improve your skin's appearance. It's also the step that gives you visible results most quickly. That's because removing those rough cells improves skin color and texture almost immediately.

Exfoliation also temporarily improves circulation, so your skin appears brighter. I think skin literally glows immediately after an exfoliating treatment. People with acne may be surprised to see that not only do their fine lines and wrinkles disappear with regular chemical exfoliation with hydroxy acids, but they have fewer pimples as well. Hydroxy acids normalize the skin cell formation and shedding process in the hair follicles. The abnormal production of skin cells is one of the factors that causes blackheads and whiteheads, the precursors of acne, to form. Within a few weeks of using a hydroxy acid, you'll notice less clogging of the pores and fewer breakouts.

Some research has shown that exfoliation also stimulates collagen production deep within the skin, but scientific proof of that benefit has still not been established. If true, it could explain why exfoliation not only reduces fine lines but appears to make skin more resilient as well.

If you choose your skin care products wisely, you can sustain the rejuvenating effects indefinitely. You can accomplish a little exfoliation when you wash your face using a cleanser that contains gentle abrasive materials such as jojoba beads or cornmeal and/or hydroxy acids. You can continue the process with moisturizer that allows hydroxy acids to remain on your skin. And you can give your skin a serious turnover boost with a treatment product that contains one or more hydroxy acids once a day or several times a week. To jump-start the process or to occasionally get a dramatic improvement, you can use an exfoliating facial. And an esthetician can safely use a more concentrated solution of hydroxy acids than are available in most treatment products for consumer use. A dermatologist can use an even more powerful glycolic acid formula to actually peel the top layer of skin.

Of all the steps in my program, exfoliation illustrates perhaps most dramatically the importance of continuing the program for the rest of your life. If you stop exfoliating your skin for even a week, you will see your skin become duller as the cells soon begin accumulating again. The only good reason to stop is if your skin becomes irritated, which we'll talk about in chapter 7, Reduce Inflammation.

AHA: A TIMELESS REMEDY

It's said that sour milk baths were the secret to Cleopatra's luminously beautiful skin. Of course, we have no idea what her skin really looked like, but if sour milk kept her youthful, it's no surprise to me. Sour milk contains an exfoliating concentration of lactic acid, one of several natural hydroxy acids. These are some-

A REVOLUTION IN SKIN CARE

AHAs have been around since ancient times. In the 1970s dermatologists were using glycolic acid for skin peels. By 1989, I had treated over six thousand patients with low concentrations of AHAs in various forms, and by 1990 I had introduced AHAs in over-the-counter products that were available to the consumer. Today glycolic acid and other AHAs are ubiquitous in skin care products, and several studies have proved their merit in reducing fine lines and wrinkles and improving hydration.

It's said that AHAs were a revolution in skin care. True, some forms of AHAs were used in ancient times, but learning how to formulate AHAs in the proper concentration and the proper pH certainly initiated an entirely new way of caring for the skin.

---

times called fruit acids, because a few of them are derived from foods. Malic or mandelic acid comes from apples. Tartaric comes from grapes. Glycolic acid comes from sugar cane.

The hydroxy acids used in skin care products are synthesized versions of those found in nature. Glycolic acid, the alpha hydroxy acid I prefer, is the smallest of the alpha hydroxy molecules and is thought to be the most active.

Moisturizers that contain alpha hydroxy acids typically contain lower concentrations than do treatment products. Estheticians can use slightly higher concentrations of AHAs, up to 30 percent in a buffered solution with an adjusted pH, in their skin care treatments. And physicians use even higher concentrations of 50 to 70 percent in a nonbuffered solution. These penetrate quite deeply and are considered skin peels. You would not want to use such a potent solution at home.

Unfortunately, the concentration of a hydroxy acid in a product is not listed on its label. Neither is the pH, which affects the potency of the acid. This is a case, again, where you have to listen to your skin and pay attention to how it reacts. If your skin becomes irritated with one product, it doesn't mean you can't benefit from a hydroxy acid. What you need to do is try another formulation. Some tingling is to be expected, but severe stinging and redness is not. Of course, using a well-known, established brand is a safety precaution.

When I first incorporated hydroxy acids in my products, there was a great deal of discussion about concentration and pH. Now, most moisturizers and treatment products sold over-the-counter contain 10 percent or less of an AHA and have a pH of 3.5 or higher. Beta hydroxy acid (BHA) concentration is usually 0.5 to 2 percent. (The lower the pH, the more irritating and possibly the more potent the hydroxy acid.) This is the concentration and pH that the Esthetics Manufacturers and Distributors Alliance recommends. They suggest limiting the use of high concentrations to 30 percent with a pH of 3 to professional estheticians. Only a physician with experience doing chemical peels should use high concentrations of chemical exfoliating agents.

Hydroxy acids work by combining with the structural lipids between the layers of the cells, creating a bigger space that loosens their attachment. In the beginning, you may notice some flakiness of your skin for a few weeks, as the exfoliating action begins to separate several layers of dead cells. If this is bothersome, you can use a clay mask to hurry the process along. You don't want to use a scrub, because it will be too irritating when combined with the hydroxy acids.

AN ALPHABET OF ACIDS

Hydroxy acids are labeled alpha or beta according to their chemical structure. The most commonly used beta hydroxy acid is salicylic acid. Its mild antiseptic qualities and exfoliating action have made it a well-known acne fighter. Some products contain a mix of AHAs and BHAs. Recently, polyhydroxy acids have been introduced. Chemically, these are made of larger molecules than the AHAs and BHAs, so they don't penetrate as deeply or as easily. Consequently, they're less irritating. The downside is that they are also less active. I favor formulations that combine more active AHAs, such as glycolic acid, with skin soothers and other anti-inflammatory ingredients to counteract irritation. And always be vigilant with sun protection when using any hydroxy acid product.

After about six or eight weeks you may see a kind of plateau in the effects of exfoliation. Your skin is becoming accustomed to the hydroxy acid, and from this point on you will be improving at a slower rate. It's a little like when you first start exercising. Let's say you're walking on a treadmill with a 5 percent elevation. If you're just starting out, it's going to be tough. But your muscles become used to it, and if you want more you're going to have to walk faster or increase the elevation. With hydroxy acids, you don't want to increase the concentration of the product you're using daily, but you may want to try it twice a day, or give yourself a weekly enzyme mask treatment. You can also see an esthetician once or twice a month for an exfoliating treatment with a higher concentra-

PEELS THAT HEAL

When forty-year-old homemaker June had a skin cancer removed from her nose, her self-confidence went with it because she was left with a terrible discolored and peeling nose. "It took two years to heal after the liquid nitrogen treatment," June explains. "First it looked like a giant blister, then it looked like a raisin. Then it finally healed, but it was dark in spots and light in spots." June was embarrassed to go out, and when she did she spent hours applying camouflaging makeup.

I gave June a series of glycolic acid peels to remove the severely hyperpigmented areas on her nose. But I didn't just treat her nose. June had blond hair and blue eyes and she had spent nearly every day of her life in the sun, and she still leads a very active outdoor life with her young daughter and son, snowboarding, doing motocross, and playing on the beach. All that sun was part of the reason she had developed the skin cancer in the first place. It had also created severe hyperpigmentation on her forehead, cheeks, and along her upper lip. The glycolic acid peels immediately improved her skin tone, but June needed to maintain that improvement with diligent sun protection and daily skin treatments with AHAs and other ingredients to combat the free radicals she is nearly constantly exposed to because of her outdoor lifestyle. She also takes supplements twice a day, and a pomegranate supplement every morning.

Two years after her first glycolic acid peels, June still

has smooth, bright skin and no sunspots or hyperpigmented areas.

"I use all the skin defenses now. The changes in my face are so dramatic. I love that I don't have to wear makeup and can just put on sunscreen and go out. I could never do that before. After the peels, there was a dramatic improvement, then with the vitamin C treatments and the daily program, my skin just kept getting better," she says with confidence.

---

tion of hydroxy acid. At some point, though, you will reach a healthy threshold. You can't go further without irritating your skin.

If you use any hydroxy acid–containing products, it's important to be especially aware of sun protection. Studies have shown that people who regularly exfoliate using either a chemical or mechanical agent tan more readily than those who don't.

Resurfacing techniques with lasers or chemical agents also remove tissue and are a kind of extreme exfoliation. There is evidence that all of the methods stimulate the production of new collagen and diminish wrinkles. You may have heard of nonablative lasers. These reduce hyperpigmentation and dilated blood vessels deep in the skin without injury to the epidermis, so they don't remove skin cells.

There are also enzymes in various masks and skin treatments that digest protein, so they are helpful in literally dissolving superficial skin cells. There are natural ones such as papain, which is derived from papaya, and bromelain, which comes from pineapple. There are also synthetic ones that are quite effective.

SHOPPING FOR AN EXFOLIATING AGENT

I know some people prefer to use all-natural ingredients, but I think with some ingredients, synthetic substances have an advantage in terms of uniformity and consistency. Although people believe that real fresh fruit is used in "all natural" products, the botanical ingredient is usually an extract. Natural extracts are standardized, so you know you are getting a specific amount of the active components. In my products with pomegranate, for example, I use a standardized extract of pomegranate. When I'm formulating a product, I use the ingredients that I think are best. For some properties, I may incorporate a natural essential oil or a standardized extract, and for others, such as glycolic acid, where uniformity is critical, I will use a synthetic form.

And some people prefer to mechanically remove the dead cells with a loofah, Buf-Puf, or scrubs and cleansers with gentle abrasive ingredients such as cornmeal, rice grains, or jojoba beads. Scrubs made with particles that have sharp edges, such as ground apricot pits, beans, and seashells, may be too abrasive, especially for those with sensitive skin.

All of these exfoliation methods work, but I think the hydroxy acids have several advantages over the others. They not only remove the dead cells, they also reduce excessive buildup of skin cells within the hair follicles. In this way, they prevent breakouts, acne, and brown spots as well as maintain a smoother skin surface. I often suggest that people with acne also use an enzyme treatment once or twice a week to gently and effectively boost the exfoliation process.

I believe that everyone over the age of twenty needs some exfoliation to counter the slowdown in cell turnover. How much you need is unique to you. Also, some people prefer to combine exfoliation with cleansing. Or, since a good hydroxy acid treatment product also contains moisturizing ingredients, they'll prefer to use a treatment product as a moisturizer. It's really a personal choice. But be careful of overprocessing your skin. If you are using a scrub or a cleanser, a moisturizer, and a treatment product that all contain one or more types of hydroxy acid every day, and your skin is red and feels tight, it's obvious that you're overdoing it. I usually suggest starting with a daily hydroxy acid treatment product, and if your skin tolerates it well, you can try increasing the exfoliation with, say, a hydroxy acid–containing cleanser. Usually, people with oily skin can tolerate this regimen quite well.

On the other hand, if your daily use of a hydroxy acid treatment is making your skin sting and feel stretched, cut back to using the treatment product three days a week, and then listen to your skin. Men who shave every day may not need as much exfoliating as women, because as they shave they remove the top layer of dead cells. However, because their skin is thicker than a woman's is, they can usually benefit from using a hydroxy acid treatment product as well. The daily exfoliation of shaving may be one reason why they tend to have fewer fine lines on their cheeks and jawline than women do.

Ingredients to Look For
Salicylic acid
Glycolic acid
Lactic acid
Jojoba beads
Papain or bromelain enzymes

SIX

Disarm Free Radicals

Whenever I ask my patients and people that I speak to around the world, "What causes aging?" they will give me a list that includes smoking, pollution, smog, sun, stress, and poor diet. Then I point out that what all these things have in common is that they all create free radicals. We need to protect ourselves from these insults in any way that we can, and we need to disarm the free radicals that are created, with antioxidants.

While free radicals are destructive in several ways, I believe that the most significant damage is done when they steal atoms from the lipids in the cell wall. Ultimately this breaks down the cell barrier, the membrane that holds the cell together and defends it. And the result is water escapes from the cell, leading to irreparable injury and premature cell death. By keeping the skin flooded with antioxidants, much of this damage—and water loss—is prevented.

Skin is wondrously efficient at self-repair, which is a very good thing, considering it's the most environmentally damaged of all the organs in the body. Fortunately, when we're healthy and well nour-

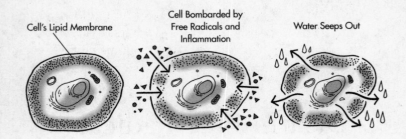

Cell's Lipid Membrane

Cell Bombarded by
Free Radicals and
Inflammation

Water Seeps Out

Free radicals and inflammation damage the cell wall, allowing water and other vital contents to escape prematurely.

ished, we have natural antioxidant enzymes that disarm free radicals before they cause so much trouble. You may not have heard of these enzymes, with unwieldy names like superoxide dismutase and glutathione peroxidase, but keeping a robust supply is one reason why it's important for you to get enough of the minerals from which they are made, such as copper, zinc, and selenium.

Another source of antioxidants is foods. The antioxidant vitamins C, E, and beta-carotene are abundant in fruits and vegetables, so if you eat these foods and take supplements, you can help keep the free radicals in your body in check. The skin, however—especially the topmost layers, which are the first defense against environmental assaults—needs extra help, which is why I think it's so important to apply antioxidants to the skin.

Each cell of your body sustains about a thousand hits each day by free radicals generated by its own metabolism. That's not counting the immeasurable hits that occur as a result of exposure to smoke and pollution, a hard workout, and the most significant factor of all—ultraviolet radiation from the sun. When your ability to defend against free radicals is weak—and some aging researchers think your defenses weaken as you grow older—or when there are just too many to contend with, a situation occurs that biologists call *oxidative stress*. In that state the free radicals that aren't quickly disarmed begin a relentless search for the atoms that will make them complete. And a prime target of their search are the lipids that form the walls of your cells. As those lipids are bombarded, the contents of the cell—namely water—escape. A plentiful supply of fatty acids can help replenish the lipids that are broken down, but perhaps even that is inadequate.

The destruction that accompanies oxidative stress affects all of the body's cells, not just those in the skin. Free radicals target cells' energy centers, the mitochondria, for instance. And when the mitochondria are attacked, they churn out even more of the loose molecules. Ultimately, free radicals can damage the genetic material, the DNA, in cells, which is one of the factors that can trigger cancer.

If aging were solely the result of free radical damage, then we might be able to extend life by supplying enough antioxidants to keep the scale tipped in favor of defense. Since the late 1950s, when the free radical theory of aging was first proposed, many experiments have shown that antioxidants help animals live longer, but results of these studies are conflicting.

YOUR BEST DEFENSE

Free radical damage is one aging factor that you can do something about. You can be sure your body is supplied with sufficient natural antioxidants by eating foods that contain them and taking supplements. You can literally boost your skin's defenses by applying antioxidants topically. I was one of the first to incorporate antioxidants into skin care, and by 1992 they were in every Murad product. Today antioxidants are as ubiquitous in skin care treatment products as hydroxy acids. The early days of skepticism have passed as countless studies have proven that antioxidants applied to the skin's surface offer protection from sun damage and stimulate collagen production. There is also scientific evidence that taking antioxidants internally in supplements increase the level of antioxidants in the skin.

People talk about antioxidants as if they are uniform. They're not. Think about antibiotics: each one targets a different group of similar bacteria. The same is true of antioxidants. While they're active throughout the body, including the skin, different ones seem to have a preference for certain organs. Ginkgo biloba, for instance, appears to be most effective in the brain. Superoxide dismutase works best within blood vessels. The flavonoids are helpful in the liver. Vitamin C works well within the bladder: it's excreted in the urine, so as the urine pools in the bladder, the bladder lining is bathed in the antioxidant. Vitamin A is especially effective on cells in the lungs and skin. Polyphenols are quite active in the skin.

There's some evidence that free radical damage has a certain rhythm. The damage free radicals do to the lipid membranes of the cells tend to accumulate during the day, reaching a peak at about bedtime. That's why I suggest using an antioxidant treatment product and taking an antioxidant supplement morning and night. If you apply antioxidants topically, then during the night when you're at rest and you are not exposed to the sun, the antioxidants have a great opportunity to do their job unimpeded. I think it's important to take antioxidant supplements twice a day, in the morning and at night, so that there is a constant supply circulating in the bloodstream.

So let's take a look at the antioxidants that I believe are most important to the skin, the only organ that allows us to see visible proof that countering free radical damage can reverse some of the changes of aging.

There are probably hundreds if not thousands of antioxidants that curtail free radicals at different levels. This is not meant to be an exhaustive list, but rather a discussion of the antioxidants that

I feel are effective when applied to the skin's surface and that are widely available in skin care products and in supplements.

VITAMIN C

Unlike many other animals, humans are not able to make their own ascorbate, or vitamin C, but must obtain it through food. A constant supply is needed because vitamin C doesn't linger too long in the tissues, and it's continually excreted in the urine.

Vitamin C is a multitasker in the skin. In the epidermis, where there is five times more vitamin C than in the deeper skin layers, it performs several functions. It helps prevent water loss and therefore maintains the skin's barrier function. It is involved in collagen and elastin building. And it deactivates the unstable free radicals before they can cause too much damage. There is also increasing evidence that vitamin C shields the skin from the sun's burning rays, especially when it's applied in high concentrations or combined with vitamin E, sunscreens, and skin soothers.

There's a limit to how much vitamin C the body will absorb from food. So when Duke University and University of Wisconsin researchers discovered that it was possible to bypass the body and deliver the nutrient directly to the skin, increasing its vitamin C content by about twenty times, dermatologists all over the world realized that the skin could literally be fed vitamin C from the outside.

Today, nearly a decade after this discovery was made, we have learned much more about topical preparations of vitamin C. Cosmetic chemists now know that the percentage and type of vitamin C used makes a difference and so does the pH of the product. I've spent many years working with cosmetic chemists to develop an over-the-counter, highly concentrated, stable vitamin C product that people can easily use at home.

Vitamin C is actually quite delicate. It is water soluble, but when mixed with water and exposed to oxygen it isn't able to maintain its antioxidant activity. Also, vitamin C rapidly disintegrates when exposed to light. After much painstaking research, I developed and patented a technology that uses a highly concentrated form of vitamin C in a water-free lotion. It's a rich, soothing cream that can deliver pure vitamin C to the upper layers of the skin without irritation and in consistently high amounts. Over the years since this discovery, we've learned that repeated use of vitamin C is best, because applying it every day helps build a reservoir of vitamin C in the skin.

There are also "mix and use" products that involve mixing vitamin C into a base or vehicle and applying it immediately while the vitamin C is still active. I think these products are quite useful, especially for higher concentrations of vitamin C. Estheticians at spas and physicians can use a specially formulated infusion treatment that delivers even higher concentrations of vitamin C. The irritation potential of such high concentrations of vitamin C is eliminated by including skin soothers (see chapter 7, Reduce Inflammation) and an emollient in the formula.

Without anti-inflammatory agents, a vitamin C product might even be counterproductive, since inflammation creates free radicals. In some cases, a vitamin C product can be so irritating that it causes the skin to swell. That may make fine wrinkles disappear momentarily, but the effect doesn't last and the side effect is mild inflammation.

VITAMIN E

There are actually eight different types of molecules that fall under the vitamin E umbrella. They all contain the same elements, but their molecular shapes vary so that they can fit different receptors on cells. All of them are attracted to lipids, such as those in the walls of cells, which makes them important players in enhancing the cells' ability to hold water, and all of them are fat soluble.

Vitamin E is unique in many ways, one of which is the multiple roles it plays. It is, of course, a potent antioxidant. But it's also a marvelous emollient, preventing transepidermal water loss, so it's often included in moisturizing products. And it is a soothing anti-inflammatory, which you'll learn more about in the next chapter. Vitamin E is also stable in water, which makes it easier to use in products. In fact, it's so stable that it's often used in cosmetics to preserve the integrity of the other ingredients.

An active antioxidant form of vitamin E is alpha-tocopherol, and it is abundant in the lower levels of the stratum corneum, where vitamin C levels tend to be quite low, and in lesser amounts in the deeper layers of the skin. Despite the fact that your body attempts to keep the stratum corneum well fortified with vitamin E by continuously delivering tocopherol to the surface of the skin in sebum, there never seems to be enough. Studies show that a single, strong blast of sunlight immediately destroys half of whatever tocopherol is there. Also, considering the fact that we are all trying to eat less oil in our foods, it's not so easy to consume enough vitamin E in food to keep up with the demand for its antioxidant power.

Both vitamins C and E are destroyed by sunlight, but vitamin E is also especially vulnerable to depletion by ozone in the atmosphere. That's another reason why it is so important to keep the upper layers of the skin saturated with alpha-tocopherol.

Countless studies have been published documenting the effect of topical vitamin E in reducing free radical damage. In one, free radical formation was tracked after exposure to cigarette smoke. The number of free radicals gradually increased to reach a peak twenty-four hours after the initial blast of smoke hit the skin. When the test was repeated following application of vitamin E, the amount of free radicals was cut nearly in half.

Over the past two decades many studies have been done in animals and humans showing that when vitamin E is used before sun exposure, there is less redness and swelling of the skin, less destruction of lipids, and fewer sunburn cells. Some studies have shown that vitamin E's anti-inflammatory action can also kick in to reduce redness after sun exposure. When both vitamin C and E are combined, there is even more sun protection. However, there must be a high concentration of both vitamins in the skin to withstand the barrage of free radicals created by sunlight.

Vitamins C and E have an unusual relationship. Vitamin E has the unique ability to be recycled. Vitamin C, as it happens, is needed for this regeneration to occur. For this reason, I suggest looking for both antioxidants in most skin care products to help fight free radicals.

POLYPHENOLS

There's been an explosion in research documenting the health benefits of natural antioxidants in polyphenols when used topically or taken internally. Polyphenols are phytochemicals, which is just a fancy way of saying chemicals from plants. Polyphenols include very powerful antioxidants called flavonoids, which are molecules that can be quite complex, such as quercetin, which is found in green tea and grapes. There are simple ones, too, such as catechins, which are also found in tea. You'll be learning more about one of the most potent flavonoids—ellagic acid—in chapter 9. Flavonoids are not only effective scavengers of free radicals on their own, they also stimulate an increase in the body's own built-in antioxidant, glutathione.

At one time the power of flavonoids was so widely recognized that as a group they were called vitamin F, but they were never considered essential nutrients. That view may be changing now as study after study throughout the world is showing how flavonoids strengthen and repair cells and organs throughout the body. Recently, there's been a resurgence in interest in using some flavonoids topically to both fight free radicals in the epidermis and reduce inflammation.

I include standardized extracts of green tea, grape seed, and pomegranate in many of my products primarily for their antioxidant powers. But like many other phytochemicals, these are truly multipurpose agents. Grape seed extract, for instance, not only disarms free radicals; studies have shown that it also reinforces the structural fibers of the skin, collagen and elastin. And, as a bonus, grape seed is a source of essential fatty acids.

COENZYME Q 10

There are scores of other antioxidants that are taken orally or used topically to disarm free radicals. For example, ubiquinone, or coenzyme Q 10, has received a great deal of attention as an antioxidant that may prevent heart disease. It's also an active ingredient in a few skin care lines. Ubiquinone is a fat-soluble antioxidant like vitamin E. Ubiquinone is stored in cell walls, where it reacts with and disarms free radicals when the lipid membrane is under attack. It's also one of the few antioxidants that is in the mitochondria, the cells' energy factories.

When we ingest food, it goes through a process called the Krebs cycle and is ultimately converted to energy called ATP. The final step before the production of ATP is the breakdown of another chemical called ADP, a process that is under the direction of ubiquinone. This may explain how ubiquinone affects people's energy levels. For instance, in my experience, I am capable of doing more exercise if I've taken a coenzyme Q 10 supplement a half hour before my workout. Another antioxidant purported to have this effect is alpha lipoic acid. Coenzyme Q 10 is especially prevalent in the epidermis, but by the time the skin cells die and reach the stratum corneum, there is little ubiquinone left to contribute to skin's defenses. Animal studies have shown that it may protect the skin from sun damage by suppressing the production of the collagen-destroying enzyme collagenase.

The body can make its own ubiquinone, but some studies indicate that when there's less than optimal production, the deficiency contributes to heart disease. This antioxidant protects all of the body's cells, but the heart appears to need the biggest supply. There is evidence that when used topically it penetrates between the cells. I recommend it mostly as a supplement.

SHOPPING FOR INGREDIENTS

There are so many antioxidants available now in skin treatment products that you can easily find a cleanser, toner, and moisturizer that contain them. From a treatment perspective, though, the "treat and repair" step in your daily regimen is the point at which you want to saturate your skin with the most intense concentration of antioxidants, particularly vitamin C. The challenge is to find a vitamin C treatment that is stable.

Vitamin C is very sensitive to the light, so clear solutions that have turned brownish have lost some potency. Some solutions come in dark glass containers to help protect the vitamin C from the light. These must also be stored in a cool, dry place, since heat also deactivates vitamin C. It is most stable in a solution with a very low pH, which can be quite irritating, so if you do use one of the liquid vitamin C products, you may find that you also need to

VITAMIN C INTENSIVE

Like so many of my patients, Sylvia came to me for one reason and finished her treatment not only with her skin condition resolved—in her case, adult acne—but with brighter, more youthful-looking skin.

"I'd been taking care of my skin well, I thought. I had a daily regimen of cleansing, toning, and moisturizing, and I had regular facials," says thirty-seven-year-old Sylvia. "I assumed the sudden breakouts on my neck and alongside my chin were caused by stress. I love my new job, but the transition from being a staff nurse to working as an educator for a health care company was a challenge. Still, after using some over-the-counter acne treatments with no improvement, I decided it was time to see a dermatologist."

Sylvia had noticed fine lines at the corners of her eyes and across her forehead, but it was the pimples and cysts that troubled her the most.

After three weeks of following the acne program and taking the supplements, Sylvia's skin began to clear. During the "active" phase of her treatment, Sylvia also gave herself weekly vitamin C infusion treatments. At three weeks, she was put on the oily skin program and continued the weekly vitamin C infusion treatments for another three weeks.

"My acne has never come back, except for a few minor breakouts right before my period," Sylvia says.

What she didn't expect was the overall improvement in her skin. "My skin became so much smoother," she says. "All my friends tell me, 'Your skin looks so good.'"

---

use another product, such as a moisturizer, to counter the irritation with skin soothers.

Pure vitamin C is most active and least irritating when it is in a formula that contains no water. There are forms of ascorbic acid, such as ascorbyl palmitate, that can add some antioxidant power to creams and lotions. However, for maximum benefit, pure vitamin C is best. In order to make it available in a stable form, I've formulated it in a silicone vehicle that contains no water at all. This provides maximum antioxidant potency and stability with minimal irritation.

Ingredients to Look For
Vitamin C (ascorbic acid, magnesium ascorbyl phosphate, ascorbyl palmitate)
Vitamin E
Grape seed extract
Green tea
Fruit extracts (orange, kiwi, grapefruit)
Pomegranate (ellagic acid)

Supplements
Murad Daily Renewal Complex Antioxidant Supplement
Coenzyme Q 10
Multivitamin

SEVEN

Reduce Inflammation

The hot topic in medicine since the 1980s is inflammation, and research findings about this powerful force are now making headlines in the medical press almost every day. Inflammation has been linked to countless conditions from Alzheimer's disease to diabetes to heart disease. And, yes, even wrinkles.

Inflammation is really a sign that the body is attempting to protect itself from injury or invasion. Blood vessels dilate to rush nutrients, oxygen, water, and other defensive cells to the area. That's why an inflamed area appears red and swollen. The increased blood supply also makes the skin feel warm. However, there's a downside to all this activity, especially if it's sustained for a long period of time. The various body chemicals involved in the inflammatory process ultimately have a destructive effect on cells and create an excessive amount of free radicals, which all contribute to water loss.

SUNBURN:
AN INSIDE-OUT LOOK AT INFLAMMATION

Skin is a visible indicator of health, and that makes it a good subject for studying health-threatening responses such as inflammation. Certainly, one of the most obvious examples of the inflammatory process at work is sunburn. Of course, you no longer go in the sun without adequate protection, but if you were a sun worshiper, you may recall when you baked by the pool or in your backyard with only a slather of baby oil between your tender skin and the sun's burning UVB rays.

Several hours later, after you took a shower, you noticed your skin gradually becoming more and more red. If you had really overdone it, you may have felt your whole body heat up, and your skin felt tender to the touch. You may have even had a fever and chills.

Exposure to ultraviolet radiation triggers a panoply of cellular defenses under the skin. The blast of UVB rays attacks the living cells of the epidermis. The UVA rays, which are longer and penetrate deeper, attack the structures within the dermis, including the walls of the blood vessels. Very quickly, before the skin even begins to turn red, the blood vessels dilate to deliver more oxygen and defensive white blood cells to the dermis and the epidermis. The side effect of this biological strategy is that the cells of the blood vessels become larger and the walls become thinner. Water from the bloodstream leaks through them and into the surrounding tissue, causing swelling within the hour. The cells of the blood vessel walls also release inflammatory proteins called cytokines.

Despite these defensive efforts, there is cell death and destruction throughout the skin that's been exposed to the sun. Damaged skin cells, called *sunburn cells,* appear within the epidermis, especially near the bottom portion where cells are formed. And

Langerhans' cells—those critical immune system cells—are nearly completely wiped out within twenty-four hours.

Scientists who study inflammation have done some interesting experiments to document the changes that occur in sunburned skin. In some studies they create blisters on sunburned skin. The fluid that fills the blister comes from deep within the skin and can be sampled by researchers for analysis. As a result of some of these experiments, it's known that various chemicals that regulate inflammation peak within four to eight hours of exposure to ultraviolet light. These chemicals include various interleukins, prostaglandins, an acid known as 12-HETE (12-hydroxyeicosatetraenoic acid), and arachidonic acid.

This laundry list of chemicals is important to you for one reason—they are indicators that the lipids of the skin cell walls are being destroyed. The water loss and the release of collagen- and elastin-destroying enzymes that follow are ultimately responsible for the visible signs of aging that you want to reverse and prevent. These chemicals are evidence of what is known as an *inflammatory cascade*. It is easily triggered by sunburn, as you've just learned, but it can also result from any kind of inflammation, even that caused by chronic stress. In sunburn, this cascade is believed to last about twenty-four hours, but not a lot is known about the duration of inflammation triggered by other forces, such as irritation from harsh skin treatments or pollution or stress.

The really bad news about the release of these inflammatory regulators is that they don't confine themselves to the skin but appear to have a ripple effect throughout the body. Cytokines, for instance, are secreted by cells and travel in the bloodstream to distant sites, forming a sticky texture to the inside of the blood vessel wall as they go. Ultimately this attracts fat-grabbing cells that form plaque. The plaque then goes through a series of chemical changes that may eventually create a clot, impede blood flow and cause a heart attack, stroke, phlebitis and other serious conditions.

In the bones, cytokines speed the rate of bone loss. And when they're secreted by fat cells, cytokines diminish the body's ability to use insulin. This may explain why obesity is linked to diabetes. Researchers have also discovered that when overweight people lose weight, the level of a marker of inflammation in their blood called C-reactive protein decreases. In the skin, cytokines may affect the movement of immune cells called T cells to areas of inflammation and may contribute to chronic skin conditions such as psoriasis.

The most important reason to have at least a passing awareness of the inflammatory cascade is that you can stop it at several points, reducing the potential damage to the cells of your vital organs, including your skin. Aspirin, for instance, inhibits the enzyme cyclo-oxygenase, which is released during the cascade. This is believed to be one of the reasons why a daily dose of baby aspirin prevents heart disease. Eating fish and taking omega-3 fatty acid supplements help combat the harmful type of eicosanoids that perpetuate inflammation.

Inflammation is important for another reason: it is a major cause of free radical formation. And as you learned in the previous section, free radicals lead the attack on lipids in the cell walls, which leads to water loss. So with sunburn, for instance, you have destruction of the cells with a direct hit of radiation and you get more destruction from the free radicals that are created in the process. Free radicals are both a by-product of inflammation and a source of inflammation.

Countering inflammation is most important when you're young, because this is when the inflammatory response is most active. Not only are your cells most vigilant at this time, but there are many years ahead of you during which the damage will accumulate. So when you read that most of the sun damage that will cause you wrinkles after fifty occurred when you were in your

CHRONIC INFLAMMATION

At sixty-seven, Susan continues to work full-time as a makeup artist for films and television. "When you're in the business, you take care of everyone else's skin but your own," says Susan. She groans about the twelve to fourteen hours a day on the set and jokes, "You're lucky to just wash your face in the morning and get out the door. At night, I'd put a little cold cream on my face and that was it."

As a young woman, Susan was a surfer, spending hours every day on the beaches of Southern California. The cumulative inflammation from the daily doses of ultraviolet radiation when she was very young combined with the years of neglect while she was working on one movie set after another had ravaged Susan's skin.

"I've had skin cancer removed from my face and a melanoma taken off my shoulder. I still have those little red capillaries around my nose and on my cheeks, but it's this dry, crinkly texture of my skin that really bothers me. I once had the most beautiful, very fair Irish/English complexion. But that was a long time ago. I'm concerned about the wrinkles, but I can't afford a major face-lift," Susan says.

My main objective in helping Susan was replenishing her skin's water supply by putting her on the Dry Skin Program with the optional glycolic acid evening treatment and weekly vitamin C infusion treatments. She also started taking the supplements that are part of the internal Dry Skin Program. Once the excessive layers of dead cells were gone, the anti-inflammatory ingredients, the antioxidants, collagen builders, and hydrators could penetrate and begin the repair work.

To Susan's surprise, doing all four steps plus the optional treatment took just a few minutes more than washing her face and putting on cold cream. And the weekly infusion treatments she did at home, which did take twenty minutes or so, forced her to be still and relax.

After five weeks on the Dry Skin Program, Susan said, "I thought I needed a deep peel, but my skin just glows and the texture is so much smoother. It's like my skin is being nourished. The pores seem smaller, and the flakiness has completely gone away. My skin just feels nice."

---

twenties, it's not just that you might have spent more days on the beach, but that in your twenties your skin was more reactive.

Protecting yourself from the sun is the most obvious step in reducing inflammation, and you'll learn more about how to minimize radiation damage in the next section. But you can also interfere with inflammation internally with anti-inflammatory and antioxidant supplements. And you can stop it—and prevent transepidermal water loss—by using anti-inflammatory agents externally.

SHOPPING FOR SKIN SOOTHERS

When the skin is severely inflamed, say in reaction to a strong irritant or a side effect of an allergy, potent anti-inflammatory drugs like cortisone are prescribed. But for countering everyday sources of inflammation, I've found natural botanicals to be very effective skin soothers. Some cause the blood vessels to constrict, counter-

acting the dilation that occurs with inflammation. Some interrupt
the inflammatory cascade before the arachidonic acid can form
the pro-inflammatory molecules.

Allantoin, which comes from comfrey root, is ubiquitous in
products from hand lotions to aftershave lotions because it's such
a marvelous skin soother. It's also thought to stimulate new tissue
growth. Panthenol, a vitamin B, also has a duel function: along
with countering inflammation, it is also a humectant that attracts
and holds water in skin.

There are many botanicals that are wonderful skin soothers.
Chamomile (*Anthemis nobilis*) is one of the most well known. It
contains a potent chemical called bisabolol that interrupts the
inflammatory cascade. Licorice root (glycyrrhizinate) also interferes with the inflammatory cascade. Orange extract, which also
contains vitamin C, arnica, and willow herb (*Epilobium angusti-
folium*), are other commonly used natural anti-inflammatories.
The sap from the aloe vera leaf is not only a wonderful hydrating
botanical, it's also an anti-inflammatory that seems to boost the
activity of other skin soothers.

Zinc, a trace mineral, is truly a workhorse ingredient. It protects the skin from ultraviolet light and other irritants and infection from bacteria and fungi. It promotes collagen building,
enhances the effects of vitamins A and E, and soothes irritation,
whether it's caused by too much sun or acne.

Curcumin, the substance that gives the spice turmeric its yellow color, is best known as a curry ingredient, but it has long been
used as a home remedy in poultices to relieve pain and inflammation. There is a reason it's so effective. Curcumin inhibits production of a type of white blood cell that triggers inflammation, and
it blocks formation of one of the chemicals in the inflammatory
cascade. Curcumin, like many anti-inflammatory agents, is also
an antioxidant.

Curcumin is so powerful that it may help squelch the severe

skin problems that follow radiation. Oncologists found that lab animals fed curcumin before radiation therapy didn't develop the burns and blisters that are so common with this treatment. As a result, the research team that did this experiment recommended that cancer patients undergoing radiation therapy consider eating curry.

Topical antioxidants, such as pomegranate and vitamins C and E, also reduce inflammation by curtailing free radicals. One reason vitamin E is thought to be such a potent anti-inflammatory is that it not only disarms free radicals but also appears to stop the release of arachidonic acid from lipids in the cell walls. Not only that, vitamin E inhibits the formation of prostaglandins and the destructive enzyme cyclo-oxygenase as well.

Ingredients to Look For
Arnica
Licorice (glycyrrhizinate)
Aloe vera
Curcumin (*Cucurma longa*)
Chamomile (*Anthemis nobilis*)
Other soothing botanicals: cucumber, peach, lavender, Canadian willow herb, calendula, and meadowsweet
Panthenol
Allantoin
Zinc

Supplements
Murad Daily Renewal Complex Antioxidant Supplement

EIGHT

Repair Collagen

Repairing the collagen and elastin fibers that give skin its resiliency and strength is part defense, part offense. Defending the dermis, which contains the fibers and the fibroblasts that make them, from inflammation and free radicals is essential, since these are the destructive forces that cause the release of collagenase and elastase, the enzymes that literally chew up the fibers. Maintaining the lipid membranes of the fibroblasts is important, too, so that the fiber factories stay healthy and up to doing their job. Then, the next and last challenge is self-repair, rebuilding what has been injured or destroyed. There is increasing evidence that the fibroblasts can be prodded into increasing collagen and elastin production. That, in fact, is what happens when a wound heals.

WHY A FACE-LIFT ISN'T ENOUGH

As you'll recall from chapter 2, collagen fibers bundled together in an orderly way give structure and strength to the skin. The elastin

gives skin its stretch and resiliency. Over time and with sun damage, the bundles of collagen become disorderly and stiff. The collagen fibers become bent and bind to each other in a tangled
mass. The elastin fibers become hard and lose their stretch.
Fibroblasts die and collagen and elastin production slows.

At the same time this is happening to the collagen and elastin,
the fabric of the skin itself has become thinner, and some of the
bones of the skull shrink. Add the pull of gravity to this situation
and you get sags and bags, especially in areas where the underlying fat has loosened and folded over on itself. This slippage is
what causes the deep folds that extend down from either side of
the nose to the corners of the mouth or in the sagging jowls under
the chin and along the jawline.

Of course, the quick fix for skin that's become too big for
itself is a deep face-lift, in which the fat and tissues underlying
the skin are lifted and tacked down where—or nearly where—
they used to be, and the skin is lifted and pulled taut. One reason why repositioning the skin and underlying tissues can only
approximate what you looked like when you were younger is
that the quality of your skin isn't any younger. For most people,
it's still middle-aged at best. The collagen and elastin fibers are
unchanged. And the older a person is and the more sun damage
they've had, the more likely it is that the ground substance of
the dermis is lacking in nutrients and water. Given this environment, collagen and elastin production continues its downward
spiral.

Quick fixes like deep peels that aim to improve skin texture
and color are called *resurfacing techniques*. They are rejuvenating
because if they are deep enough, they affect the collagen and
elastin. Regardless of how it's done, with a laser, chemicals, or an
abrading instrument, the skin is injured in a very controlled way.
In response to the injury, the fibroblasts are jolted into action.
Your built-in survival mechanisms go into overdrive, and your

fibroblasts start churning out collagen and elastin molecules, among other things, to close or "heal" the wound.

Once the healing is complete, though, the skin continues to age at the same pace as before the resurfacing. True, you're starting off from a much better foundation, but you haven't done anything to improve the skin's health or function.

REJUVENATING TOOLS

I think many of the tools that dermatologists and plastic surgeons have today can be helpful in improving many of the changes related to aging and sun damage. Still, understanding the limitations of some of these procedures as well as the benefits will help you have realistic expectations. For instance, a face-lift will tighten skin. A deep face-lift will reposition the underlying tissues as well as tighten the skin. Resurfacing techniques remove the fine lines and hyperpigmented areas, but removing the top layers of skin will not alter deep wrinkles. Botox (botulinum toxin) injections temporarily paralyze muscles, so you are unable to contract them, giving the illusion of smoother skin. Wrinkle fillers like collagen, fat, and hyaluronic acid gel temporarily plump the depression of a fine line or scar or a hollow area, again giving the impression of smoothness or fullness. All of these measures help you appear more youthful. You can enhance their benefits by following my program and improving your skin's texture and resilience.

SUPPLY THE SKIN WITH RAW MATERIALS

What we've learned from watching how wounds heal, including those created by the controlled injury of a laser or chemical peel, is that several raw materials are needed for collagen and elastin production. These include vitamins A, B, and C, zinc, and copper. These nutrients are in most foods you eat, though supplements will guarantee you a full supply.

From animal studies we've learned that other nutrients can also increase the efficiency of wound healing. For instance, amino acids, building blocks of the protein in connective tissue, promote wound healing. It is believed that glucosamine sulfate also encourages the manufacture of connective tissue, inhibits the enzymes that break it down, and has some anti-inflammatory actions.

Connective tissue throughout the body literally connects tissues to each other. Joints and tendons are connective tissue. Muscle fibers are connective tissue. And, of course, the dermis of the skin is connective tissue. Though the shape and form of connective tissue varies depending on its location and function, it all contains collagen and elastin, fibroblasts, and the ground substance that surrounds them. As I mentioned earlier, you can think of the dermis as a mud roof: the straw fibers are the collagen and elastin, and the mud holding it all together is the ground substance, which is mostly water.

Studies of how connective tissue functions in one area and what affects its development give us important clues as to what influences connective tissue repair and maintenance in another area. When I began developing the concept that I call Internal Skin Care, researching the building blocks of skin and the raw materials needed by the fibroblasts in the dermis, I found that some of the most exciting discoveries involved the connective tissues of cartilage of the joints. Cartilage, like skin, is largely water. And many people with joint problems in which cartilage is damaged, such as arthritis, take glucosamine supplements for pain relief. Glucosamine is one building block of connective tissue. It is made by the body and is involved in the manufacture of GAGs, which, as it turns out, are abundant in cartilage and skin.

Wound-healing experiments have provided more evidence that The Water Principle works. These studies show that glucosamine stimulates the fibroblasts to produce hyaluronic acid is a major water-holding molecule in GAGs. In fact, recent studies have shown that when glucosamine is taken by mouth in the first days after surgery, the wound heals more quickly and with less scarring. Chondroitin is another substance in glycosaminoglycans. Much less is known about chondroitin, but it's thought to inhibit a destructive enzyme.

Until two years ago, studies on the effect of glucosamine and cartilage breakdown in people with arthritis were conflicting. Some research found that people got better, others didn't. And there were questions about whether glucosamine and chondroitin could actually be absorbed by the body. Recently Canadian researchers concluded a three-year study involving more than two hundred people with arthritis of the knee. Half took glucosamine every day for three years and the other half took a fake pill, though none of the volunteers knew which tablet they were taking. The researchers published their surprising findings in the prestigious medical journal the *Lancet*. The 106 people who took the placebo had progression of their disease. Their symptoms worsened slightly. And X rays of their knees showed that the joint space between the two leg bones became smaller. Those who took glucosamine, however, had little if any progression of joint-space narrowing, and 20 to 25 percent of them had less pain.

MAKE COLLAGEN BETTER

It seemed to me that all the research done in wound healing, connective tissue, and cartilage pointed in one direction: Supply the body with raw materials—such as amino acids, vitamins, minerals, *and* glucosamine—and collagen production improves. After all, the components of cartilage and skin are very similar. Both need hyaluronic acid to hold on to water and insure the quality and quantity of GAGs which, in turn, nourish the cells that make collagen and elastin.

I didn't know if it was possible to increase the efficiency of the fibroblasts by providing the body with more raw materials, but I suspected that it was. If you have a fibroblast that can produce enough protein fibers to form a bundle of collagen in a certain period of time, then, I thought, providing enough raw materials to make three bundles should yield at least one. So I developed and patented a formula called Youth Builder that could be taken internally and included not just glucosamine but a balance of all the nutrients needed to build collagen and elastin. (You can see the exact formula in the appendix.) By taking the supplement you are helping the fibers that are there to last longer and you're encouraging new ones to form and perhaps at a faster rate than before.

The fibroblast is like a plant that produces a fruit or a flower. The ground substance is the soil. The ground substance needs water along with the other nutrients to nourish the plant. Giving that ground substance certain amino acids, vitamins, minerals, and glucosamine enables the fibroblasts to flourish and produce collagen and elastin molecules.

To test my concept, an independent laboratory asked seventy-three women between the ages of thirty-nine and fifty-three to participate in a study. Anyone who had chemical peels or had been using Retin-A, both of which affect collagen production, was not included. The women put nothing on their skin—no moisturizers, special cleansers, foundations, or sunscreens—for one week. The only thing they could do to their skin was to cleanse it with soap, and they all used the same one. After a week, the women came into the laboratory and spent about an hour in a very controlled environment. Then technicians took various measurements of the number, length,.and depth of their fine lines or crow's-feet, the bounce and elasticity of the skin of their cheeks, and the amount of water in their stratum corneum.

After all these baseline tests were done, the women began taking the Youth Builder supplement twice a day. Another group went through the same process but didn't take Youth Builder.

In two weeks, the tests were repeated, and the technicians taking the measurements didn't know who had taken the supplement and who had not. They found a minimal 8 percent improvement in the depth and number of their fine lines and a 10 percent increase in skin elasticity. An appreciable increase, but not nearly as remarkable as the measurements taken three weeks later. Five weeks after taking the supplements, there was a statistically significant 34 percent reduction in the depth of the wrinkles and number of lines and an 18 percent increase in the skin's bounce, indicating that the skin was softer and more yielding.

The supplement was encouraging elastin production. There was no increase in hydration of the stratum corneum, which was actually what I wanted to see. The lack of water showed me that the women had followed instructions and had not used a moisturizer. Surface hydration is important to measure, because if the women had used a moisturizer, it would have temporarily reduced fine lines and confused the study results.

The report from the independent laboratory concluded that the improvement in the skin's appearance was probably due to a change in the connective tissue. Of course, the improvement seen in the facial skin would occur in skin all over the body, on the neck, the chest, and the backs of the hands.

LIVING PROOF

Seventy-four-year-old Sue Ann is a perfect controlled study. For about twenty years she has been using hydrators, antioxidants, anti-inflammatory agents, collagen builders, and sun protection on the back of one hand and not the other. I didn't recruit Sue Ann for this unusual study, rather she unwittingly did it herself. She's an esthetician, who in the process of doing countless facials using my skin treatment products, had put them on the back of her left hand. She would then transfer them from that palette to her clients' faces.

"I often show the backs of my hands to clients," Sue Ann says. " 'Now here is a seventy-four-year-old hand.' I point to my right hand, which is wrinkled and blotchy; and then I show them the other, that has no wrinkles and not a single age spot. I tell them, as I put my two hands side by side, 'This is why I'm a believer.' "

SHOPPING FOR COLLAGEN BUILDERS

There are several ingredients that appear to boost collagen production from the outside. Vitamin C, for example, is essential to the production of healthy connective tissue, and it's known to stimulate the fibroblasts to produce collagen. What hasn't been known until recently is that topical vitamin C penetrates the skin to promote collagen production, too. And by disarming free radicals, vitamin C protects collagen from further destruction.

Alpha hydroxy acids also appear to stimulate collagen production, though the mechanism for this action isn't known.

But one of the major beauty breakthroughs is the use of vitamin A derivatives to increase collagen production. Retinol, the natural form of vitamin A, combines four wrinkle fighters in one. It's an exfoliating agent, because it increases cell turnover. It helps to build collagen. It protects the fibers from damage by blocking the action of collagen-digesting enzymes. And it is an antioxidant that combats free radicals. Furthermore, it does all this to rejuvenate the skin with far fewer side effects than tretinoin (see box below).

Although retinol appears to be most active in the epidermis, where the skin cells are developing, research has also shown that it does penetrate as far as the dermis.

Retinyl palmitate is simply a kinder, gentler form of vitamin A. It's not as active as retinol, but many people with sensitive or very dry skin who can't use retinol-containing products find they tolerate retinyl palmitate quite well. It's believed that retinyl palmitate is converted to retinol in the skin and eventually the retinol becomes retinoic acid.

THE PRESCRIPTION WRINKLE CREAM

Sixty years ago, scientists began developing synthetic forms of vitamin A called retinoids. Many have been used as drugs, and one of them—tretinoin—has proved effective for acne and wrinkles.

Topical tretinoin is available by prescription as Retin-A or Renova. Retin-A is most commonly used for acne. Renova, which is tretinoin in an emollient base, is a powerful skin rejuvenator.

Tretinoin, also known as all-trans-retinoic acid, reduces fine lines, smoothes the skin's texture, and normalizes pigmentation. Tretinoin does appear to reverse some of the signs of aging, especially those caused by sun damage.

There's no doubt that tretinoin is effective in helping skin appear and function like younger skin. Initially, though, the drug may be irritating and some people cannot tolerate it for the several weeks the skin needs to adjust. Retinol may take longer to achieve the same result, but most people don't find it as irritating as tretinoin.

Occasionally I prescribe tretinoin for aging skin, but I always emphasize in discussing the treatment with my patients that this drug addresses only one aspect of aging skin. They still need antioxidants, anti-inflammatory agents, and hydrators to defend their skin from further damage. In fact, they need these other anti-aging components—inside and out—even more to counter some of the irritation, inflammation, and drying that often accompany tretinoin use. I stress the need to always use a broad-spectrum sunscreen even on cloudy days. Tretinoin makes the skin supersensitive to sunlight, and exposure that is normally tolerated can cause severe sunburn.

Finally, women in their childbearing years must be very careful not to become pregnant while taking Accutane. Accutane, the form of retinoic acid that is taken internally, is known to cause birth defects, but the safety of any of the topical retinoids, including retinol, in pregnancy has not been established.

Ingredients to Look For
Retinol
Retinyl palmitate
Alpha hydroxy acids
Vitamin C (ascorbic acid, magnesium ascorbyl phosphate, ascorbyl palmitate)
Amino acids

Supplements
Murad Youth Builder Collagen Supplement

NINE

Protect

By now there's not a person alive in America who doesn't know that too much time in the sun causes premature aging and skin cancer. And most people are aware that the earlier that exposure begins—particularly when it causes sunburn—and the longer it goes on, the worse the damage is.

Of course you need to start immediately protecting yourself from ultraviolet radiation. By taking this protective step you are also helping to reverse sun damage. Studies have shown that by simply using sunscreen and therefore curtailing the inflammation caused by radiation, the skin can do a terrific job at self-repair.

I have a tool called a skin scanner that conveys to every person who walks through the door of my spa or my private practice the ugly, aging effects of tanning. The scanner is a special light that allows you to see the damage beneath your skin, the subclinical damage that has not yet become apparent. People can see what they will look like years down the road if they stop sunbathing today. Splotches of altered pigmentation created by impaired pigment-producing cells are shockingly obvious under the light of this viewing device. Wrinkles, even fine ones, stand out. It's a surprise to everyone to see what damage is lurking there, and most men and women who get this glimpse into their own future quickly change their habits.

Another convincing experience is the first time a person has a suspicious lesion removed from his or her face. This brush with reality usually convinces the person that tanning can have a steep price. In most cases, the lesion turns out to be normal, but the day or two of suspenseful waiting for the laboratory results can put the fear of tanning into a person.

Because ultraviolet radiation is such a powerful aging accelerator, sun protection is a crucial wrinkle fighter. Some of the damage done in the past can be repaired with proper hydration and topical and internal antioxidants, collagen-builders, and anti-inflammatory agents, but nothing can restore youth back to the skin if it's not protected from further injury.

You already know what every dermatologist and newspaper and magazine article says about preventing wrinkles and skin cancer: Apply sun protection daily, wear a hat and protective clothing, and avoid sun exposure between 11:00 A.M. and 3:00 P.M. But, if you're like most of my patients, you don't always comply with this advice. I've noticed that even after a cautionary lecture from me, people come back on follow-up visits a little more sun-damaged than before. Of course, if I hadn't delivered my usual lecture about how dangerous sun is, their skin might look even worse. But for the most part, on a scale of 0 (no worsening of sun damage) to 10 (severe sun damage), they come back one or two points above where they started. My goal is to have them return to one or two points below their starting point. And over the last twenty years, I've developed a way to make that happen. My program involves not only using topical sun protection but supplements to boost the power of the sunscreen and supply antioxidants, anti-inflammatories, and hydrating agents.

Years ago I noticed that sunscreen didn't seem to be enough. Living and practicing in Southern California, where convertible cars and nearly perfect, sunny weather prevail, even those patients who I'm sure were quite diligent about using sunscreen were still getting too much sun damage. Clearly even sunscreens have limitations, and I also understand how hard it is to reapply sunscreen every two hours or more. I knew that what was needed was continuous sun protection that wasn't affected by any outside factors like sweating, swimming, or rubbing.

Considering the research on antioxidants that was being done at the time, I began to recommend that my patients take supplements of beta-carotene and vitamin C. Now, at the time in the 1980s, researchers were finding that applying antioxidants such as vitamins C and E and beta-carotene to the skin could limit the damage done by overexposure to ultraviolet light. Presumably the antioxidants were neutralizing free radicals responsible for the inflammation. Although the antioxidants helped protect the skin, so much was needed for this benefit that there were concerns about toxicity and irritation.

Studies involving taking antioxidants internally were mixed. Some researchers were reporting that beta-carotene seemed to work, while others found that it didn't. Vitamin E wasn't especially effective even when thirteen times the recommended daily allowance was given. And beta-carotene, while it might be helpful, caused people's skin to turn an unattractive orange.

I took a different approach and began treating my patients who had severe photo damage with a combination of glycolic acid peels, antioxidant supplements, and SPF 30, broad-spectrum sunscreens. They were coming back a few weeks later with less sun damage than if they had had a glycolic acid peel alone, and they were maintaining their healthy skin. The minimal but nevertheless cumulative sun damage I had seen in the past wasn't happening.

As I studied antioxidants more, I realized that they are not all created equal and that new ones are being discovered every day. Especially interesting were the studies of polyphenols, such as the flavonoids in green tea. And among the most potent of the flavonoids is in tiny red seeds of the pomegranate.

THE POWER OF POMEGRANATE

Pomegranate contains a super antioxidant called ellagic acid, which is even more powerful than the antioxidants in green tea. According to a study in the *Journal of Agriculture and Food Chemistry,* commercially prepared pomegranate juice has three times the antioxidant activity, ounce for ounce, of red wine or green tea. The researchers attribute this to the three components of pomegranate: tannins, from the rind, and anthocyanins and ellagic acid, from the seeds.

The anti-inflammatory powers of pomegranate have been well known for eons. In ancient times, Hippocrates described the medicinal powers of this native Indian and African fruit. It was used by the Greeks to treat many inflammatory conditions from bronchitis to diarrhea. Other cultures used it to treat arteriosclerosis and asthma, even to help bone regeneration after injury.

Pomegranate also appears to be effective against viruses, destroying them on contact. And it is especially effective in protecting cells from free radical damage. Other compounds in pomegranate—the anthocyanidins—interact with ellagic acid to further boost its antioxidant potency.

The powerful antioxidants in pomegranate work by boosting the levels of glutathione, a natural antioxidant in the body that helps protect the DNA in cells from free radical damage. Glutathione is also essential in helping the body recycle hormones such as estrogen, which also protect the skin cells.

Polyphenols, such as ellagic acid, also inhibit the formation of harmful enzymes that cause cells to grow out of control. This is important in terms of cancer prevention because out-of-control cell division is a hallmark of cancer. By inhibiting specific enzymes, ellagic acid and other polyphenols regulate cell turnover and give the cell time to divide normally and form completely. Ellagic acid is also thought to strengthen the cell membrane, making it less susceptible to free radical damage and preventing water loss.

To prove that pomegranate could improve the sun protection of sunscreen, I asked an independent laboratory to test eight different sunscreen formulations—four with pomegranate extract and four without it. Adding pomegranate boosted the SPF of the formula by 20 percent. Next we tested the same formulations before and after the volunteers took a daily pomegranate supplement for five days. The SPF of all the sunscreens was boosted 25 percent on average.

As a result of these findings I altered my program a few years ago. I began asking patients to combine daily use of pomegranate and other antioxidant supplements with their daily regimen and to also use a highly concentrated topical vitamin C weekly treatment for a few weeks several times a year. I noticed even better results than I had achieved with glycolic acid peels and antioxidants.

HOW SUN HURTS

To get a complete picture of how this program will benefit your skin and prevent further sun damage, it's helpful to see the link between inflammation and the changes that you see with sun damage and age. How you react to sunlight depends on several things: how much melanin you have, how easily you tan, and how many sunburns you've had in the past. If you always burn and never tan, the sun will trigger inflammation in your skin very easily within an hour of sun exposure. Other factors can affect your response, too, such as certain genetic disorders, diseases, and many drugs, such as antibiotics and nonsteroidal anti-inflammatory agents.

The inflammatory response stimulates many biochemical reactions that ultimately damage the skin, causing photoaging. Often these reactions are the opposite of what happens in natural aging, but the change that results makes skin look old before its time. For example, skin cells may develop faster, but they aren't normal and uniform. They vary in size and shape and don't fit together neatly, so the epidermis of sun-exposed skin is actually about twice as thick as sun-protected skin.

The immune cells, called Langerhans' cells, within the skin are also affected by the sun-triggered inflammation. They're less effective, and there are fewer of them. The most serious damage occurs deep within the dermis, the layer most damaged by UVA rays. Here the processes that occur with normal aging are speeded up, too. There's an overproduction of collagen fibers, but they aren't normal. They're thick and tangled. The elastin becomes thick as well. The blood vessel walls become thick, and potentially harmful inflammatory cells cluster within them. There is also a decrease in GAGs, which means there is less water to lubricate the collagen and elastin fibers and to supply the living cells of the epidermis.

Sunlight also damages the genetic material in the developing cells, creating mutations that can lead to age spots and abnormal accumulations of scaly dark cells called sun spots or actinic keratoses, some of which will progress to skin cancer.

Also, sunlight creates free radicals that break down the lipids in the cell walls, leading to water loss and inflammation.

All in all it's not a pretty picture. Fortunately, you reverse many of these changes by simply protecting yourself from further injury. That's where sunscreens come in.

SUN AND SKIN CANCER

When UV rays bombard skin, they ultimately damage the cell's genetic material. Much of this structural damage is repaired, but when the repair mechanism is damaged or inadequate, the cells may begin to grow uncontrollably and cause a malignant tumor. Ultraviolet light is directly responsible for two types of skin cancer—basal cell carcinoma and squamous cell carcinoma. Particularly severe sunburns in childhood are thought to be key risk factors. Overexposure to sunlight is also associated with the deadly form of skin cancer, melanoma.

SUN RAYS PRIMER

There are three types of radiation in the ultraviolet spectrum of sunlight: UVA, UVB, and UVC. The rays are categorized according to their wavelength, which also determines how deeply the rays penetrate the skin.

The wavelength of UVA is the longest and these rays can penetrate the skin down to the dermis. Most UVA rays pass through the ozone layer of the atmosphere to bombard the earth and your skin.

UVB rays, the middle wavelength of the ultraviolet spectrum, are mostly filtered by the ozone layer. However, those that do reach the earth can penetrate the epidermis and permanently injure developing cells. Of course, since the ozone layer is disappearing, more and more UVB radiation is now reaching the earth than did, say, twenty years ago. According to the Skin Phototrauma Foundation, for every 1 percent decrease in ozone, there will be a compounded 2 percent increase in the UVB wavelengths that reach the earth and a 3 to 6 percent increase in the incidence of skin cancer. How much more wrinkling will result can only be imagined.

UVC rays are the shortest wavelength in the spectrum, and they are totally absorbed by the ozone layer and don't injure your skin.

UVB rays are also called "sunburn radiation" because these rays, particularly the shorter ones, cause erythema, or redness of the skin as a result of dilation of the blood vessels. Usually this redness takes at least six hours to become obvious. UVA can cause redness, too, but at about a thousand times the dose of UVB. The energy of UVA rays is much more potent than UVB, and it penetrates deep into the dermis. Even when it doesn't cause redness, UVA may be more harmful than UVB, since the dermis can't regenerate itself continually as the epidermis does.

HOW SUNSCREENS PROTECT

Sunscreens protect your skin by blocking or absorbing the sun's rays. Depending on the active ingredients in the sunscreen you use, you will protect yourself from the burning ultraviolet B (UVB) rays and the more penetrating, ultraviolet A (UVA) rays.

The growing awareness of UVA's destructive power is especially disturbing because since sunscreens were invented, we have had the ability to protect ourselves against the burning UVB rays. That, obviously, is a good thing. However, the downside is that since we're less likely to burn, there is no warning sign that we've gotten too much sun. We could stay at the beach or on the golf course much longer than we might have in the days before sunscreens, exposing our skin to huge doses of UVA. Today we have broad-spectrum sunscreens that protect against both UVA and UVB rays. A UVB-screen alone is no longer considered adequate.

SHOPPING FOR SUNSCREENS

Your first criterion for choosing one is that it be *broad spectrum*, meaning it includes ingredients that absorb or block both UVA *and* UVB rays. The product you choose may be a physical block that uses zinc oxide or titanium dioxide to reflect or scatter UVB and UVA rays rather than let them pass through to the skin. A few years ago, these mineral compounds were not often used except on the noses of lifeguards because they were white or opaque. Today, the mineral particles are usually micronized, or ground so fine that they are virtually invisible.

You can also use a product that relies on chemicals to absorb UV radiation. For example, a commonly used UVA-absorber is avobenzone or Parsol 1789. You may see it listed on the label as methoxydibenzoylmethane. Absorbers tend to be more irritating than physical blocks, so people who react to chemical sunscreens may prefer zinc or titanium dioxide only. UVA-screening ingredients include absorbers such as benzophenones. UVB-screening ingredients are predominately cinnamates.

The FDA accepted SPF in 1978 as a gauge of the effectiveness of UVB sunscreens. It's a measure of sunburn protection only, and the number indicates how much longer than normal you can be in the sun without burning. An SPF 15, which is the minimum number you should wear, means that if you normally start to turn red in ten minutes, you can stay in the sun wearing the sunscreen for two and a half hours or 150 minutes (10 minutes × 15). However, that doesn't mean you can put on a SPF 15 sunscreen in the morning and forget about it till noon. To maintain the protective coverage, you need to reapply it frequently.

In the United States, SPF numbers go to 30+, but it's important to understand that as the numbers go up, the sunscreen becomes less efficient. The increments in protection actually get smaller as the numbers increase. According to the *Harvard Health Letter*, the difference between a SPF 30 and a SPF 50 is only 1.3 percent. Also, remember that the SPF applies minimally to UVA rays. Although various labeling indications have been discussed, no universal UVA-protection scale has been accepted yet. For now, you must rely on the term broad spectrum.

You can keep out about 96 percent of the sun's rays from reaching your skin just by washing your clothes with a sun-guard product called Rayosan or by wearing clothes made of a tightly woven fabric. Of course, you need to wear a hat with a wide brim, too, to shield your face, ears, and the back of your neck from the sun. Still you must use a sunscreen on whatever skin is uncovered, like your face.

Sun blockers and absorbers to protect you from the sun aren't enough. You also want to reduce the inflammation, dehydration, and free radical formation that results from the ultraviolet light that does manage to bombard your skin and penetrate your sunscreen. Many formulas available today include vitamins C and E, both of which help boost the sunscreens' protective effects. I include the antioxidant pomegranate extract as well as grape seed extract in a biovector to keep them in the very top layer of the skin, where their defensive action is most needed. And finally, I recommend taking pomegranate extract supplements to boost your sun-protection efforts.

Although we dermatologists tend to focus on what sun does to your skin, I have always believed that your whole body is affected by a day in the sun. Think about what happens when you spend a lot of time in the sun. You not only get red, you feel lethargic and dehydrated. Research now shows, too, that your immune system becomes depressed. To help protect you from these ill effects inside and out, I believe a sunscreen must contain antioxidants, anti-inflammatory agents, and hydrators. I also believe you need supplements that include antioxidants, including pomegranate, anti-inflammatories, and hydrators.

Ingredients to Look For

You need ingredients that will absorb or block UVA and UVB rays and a pomegranate supplement to boost the protective power of your sunscreen. But still some rays will get through. That's why you need a sunscreen that is bolstered with anti-inflammatory agents, hydrating ingredients, and antioxidants.

Zinc oxide
Titanium oxide
Benzophenones
Cinnamates
Pomegranate extract

Supplements
Murad Pomphenol Sunguard Supplement

TEN

Know Your Skin

Whatever your age, there are two guiding principles underlying everything you do as part of your daily basic skin care: one is to increase its moisture content, which you've just learned about. And two is to protect the skin's barrier function. Water is what keeps the cells plump and functioning. Even after the cells die, their ability to absorb moisture continues for some time. As long as the cells are moist and fit tightly together, the barrier function of skin is assured.

Protecting the topmost layers, the stratum corneum, is essential when caring for the skin. Washing, toning, and moisturizing seem so simple and straightforward that many of us take these routine skin care steps for granted, assuming we know what we're doing and using our favorite products. I've found that as knowledgeable as many men and women are, they are often victims of misinformation. They mistakenly believe, for example, that some products will shrink pores. Or that one cleanser is as good as another. "You're just going to wash it off anyway," they may have been told. Some people also believe that the skin type they are in their thirties or fifties is the same type they were a decade earlier or when they lived in the desert or in the mountains.

People often don't realize that skin type may not only change with age, it can also change in response to a shift in the external or internal environment. Traveling to a different climate or a higher or lower altitude and seasonal shifts in temperature and humidity are the most obvious examples. But certain medications, particularly hormone replacement therapy or oral contraceptives, can affect skin type, too. So do drugs designed to get rid of wrinkles, such as Retin-A, or those used to treat acne, such as Accutane. Illness, pregnancy, and menopause cause significant changes in skin physiology. Normal/combination skin can become dry. Dry skin can become oily.

SKIN TYPING

Everyone has a unique genetic profile. No two of us are exactly alike, with the exception of identical twins. The characteristics of your skin—its color and pore size, how much hair you have and where you have it, and how much sebum and sweat coats your skin—are dictated by your genes. Your skin characteristics may be similar to your father's skin or your sister's, but there are going to be important differences. After all, the medicines you take, where you live, the stress you experience are unique to you. Even identical twins are exposed to different environmental influences. And your own skin will not be the same tomorrow as it is today.

Still, dermatologists have made some generalizations and created categories of skin types into which most people can fit themselves. The Fitzpatrick Skin Types, for example, named for Thomas Fitzpatrick, the Harvard dermatologist who established them, are based on how the skin reacts to the sun. Another dermatologist, Richard Glogau, devised a system based on visible signs of aging. I believe that the standard system based on the oil and moisture content of the skin is best because it encompasses the most important factor in skin health: its ability to hold moisture. Of course, there are conditions beyond the basic type of skin that affect its care, so I modify the basic skin types with "special concerns." These include acne, pigmentation, menopause-related changes, and sensitivity.

When people think of skin type, they typically mean how oily or dry the skin is. Oil is actually a white, fatty, sticky substance secreted by the sebaceous glands. Except for the lips and eyelids, which have no hair follicles or sweat glands, sebaceous glands empty sebum into the upper part of the hair follicle. As the oil emerges from the follicle opening, or pore, it lightly coats the skin, mixing with the structural lipids within the stratum corneum, creating a kind of protective barrier that keeps water within the layers, helping the skin stay moist and soft.

When the sebaceous glands are overactive (usually in response to hormonal stimulation), the excess sebum can make skin look shiny and feel greasy. When sebaceous glands are underactive or harsh chemicals or overzealous scrubbing remove the natural lubricant, moisture is lost and the skin becomes dry.

Using sebum and structural lipids, or oil, as primary criteria, the skin types are broadly categorized as oily, dry, or normal/combination. It is normal for pores to be more abundant on the nose and chin, and so there is more oil secreted in these areas, the so-called T-zone. There are fewer pores on the cheeks and around the eyes, so these areas normally tend to be more dry.

Having lived with your skin for a couple of decades, you don't need an expert to tell you what skin type you have. The descriptions below are meant to help you confirm your own self-assessment. Or, if you're on the borderline of one type or another, these profiles should help you decide. Keep in mind that your skin type may change with different life situations—such as pregnancy and menopause—or if you move to a more dry or humid climate, and you may need to make changes in the way you care for it. With aging—and especially for women after the hormonal shifts of menopause—most people, though certainly not all, will notice that their skin is drier.

What's Normal? The pores of your skin are medium-size. Although you may have more pores along your nose and chin, and these areas may be oilier than your cheeks and around your eyes, you are not troubled with blackheads and pimples. Your complexion is bright and it feels smooth to the touch. Your skin is usually free of blemishes and tolerates extremes in temperatures well. Your cheeks may redden in the cold, but they don't become irritated and chapped. Makeup stays where you put it and doesn't flake. Weather conditions may change your skin: it's a bit oilier when it's warm and drier when it's cool.

What's Dry? Your pores are small and fine, even across your nose and chin. You may have flaky areas where there are fewer pores, and your skin is thin over your cheeks. It may be so transparent and delicate that you can see small blood vessels beneath it, especially on your cheeks. Your skin looks smooth, but it feels rough when you run your fingertips across it. There's tightness to your skin's texture within a half hour after you wash your face with a gentle cleanser, especially when you don't use a moisturizer. That tightness may even feel uncomfortable by midday. Harsh weather—cold temperatures and wind—can make it feel even worse. You may even get red, scaly patches after being outdoors. You may notice very fine superficial lines etched on your cheeks. That's because the normal creases in the skin are more obvious when there isn't enough moisture to soften them. Moisturizing creams and lotions disappear quickly into your skin after you apply them.

In a sense, dry skin is like a dry sponge. It's rough, hard, and has little cracks in it. When the sponge is soaked in water, it becomes plump, soft, and smooth, and those little cracks disappear.

Dryness is caused by lack of either sufficient sebum or structural lipids or both. So if you have dry skin, it may be because your oil glands are not producing enough sebum, or aging has taken a toll on the production of structural lipids within and outside of your skin cells, or because you are cleansing your skin too aggressively or too often. Sometimes the wrong foundation or face powder can be drying. Whatever the reason, the lack of moisture disturbs the skin's barrier function.

THIRSTY SKIN

It's unusual that someone will have dry skin because they don't drink enough water or they're dehydrated for some other reason, but it can happen. For instance, if you're very active and perspire heavily but don't replace the fluid you lose in sweat, your skin may be dry. People who drink a lot of caffeine-containing drinks or take diuretic drugs can also become dehydrated. I encourage everyone—regardless of lifestyle, diet, or environment—to be sure they drink enough water. But I think it is just as important to take fatty acids and other supplements (see chapter 13) that enable your cells to hold on to the water that reaches them.

When dryness doesn't improve despite following the appropriate basic skin care plan for dry skin that follows or it gets worse, see your physician for a checkup. Dry skin can be a warning sign of a health problem such as a thyroid condition.

What's Oily? Your pores are noticeable, your skin looks shiny at times, and it feels oily, especially along the nose and across the forehead and chin. Your overall skin tone is likely to be sallow. When it comes to aging, you are lucky. You have far fewer lines than your friends with dry or even normal skin. As you age, deeper lines, rather than fine wrinkles, will predominate.

Your skin tolerates cold and wind very well, but hot, humid weather may make it glisten with oil. Foundation disappears after about an hour or two, and moisturizing lotions and creams absorb slowly.

It's generally assumed that people with oily skin are more prone to acne. I find that in adults acne happens in all skin types. But if you are troubled with breakouts, see below.

SPECIAL CONCERNS

Regardless of skin type, breakouts may occur and some people's skin is easily irritated. Three of the most common problems are acne, environmentally stressed skin (which I call city skin), and disease.

Acne. You may have noticed a tiny pale dot of oil in your pores. Nearly everyone can see this along the sides of the nose, for instance. When that trapped sebum is exposed to the air, it turns black. Blackheads, or *comedones,* and whiteheads surface in areas where there are more oil glands, such as the sides of the nose and the middle of the chin. These breakouts can occur at any time, but they are especially common in women in the days before menstruation begins when estrogen levels are low and there is more male hormone, or androgen, in circulation.

When that oil mixes with dead skin cells and harbors bacteria, you get red, inflamed breakouts. That is acne. And despite what you have heard, oil or sebum alone doesn't cause it. Nor is acne a "teenage" problem.

Adults who never had trouble with breakouts during their teenage years can still develop acne later in life. When you're under stress, your body is producing more adrenaline or epinephrine. The same glands that produce these hormones also produce dehydroepiandrosterone (DHEA), which stimulates the sebaceous glands in the skin to produce more sebum. Women going through menopause sometimes develop acne because of the hormonal imbalance that occurs as a result of the decrease in estrogen. There is more of the male hormone androgen circulating than the female hormone, and androgen stimulates sebaceous gland activity. Excess sebum is one of the conditions that contribute to acne.

The typical acne lesion is raised, red, and sometimes even feels lumpy. In extreme cases, a cyst is formed that can lead to scarring. Most manufacturers of makeup and skin treatment products avoid ingredients known to be *comedogenic*, or known to cause comedones, but still some products can contribute to acne, as can certain drugs. If you are troubled with persistent or severe breakouts, see a dermatologist, who can do the necessary evaluation to determine the cause and prescribe the appropriate medications. An esthetician may also be of help to you with deep cleansing treatments and facials and alert you to any change for the worse that might require a dermatologist's care.

But sebum alone doesn't cause acne, so modifying oil production alone won't cure it. Therefore, I suggest following the regimen that addresses your skin type and then adding to it products that address the acne. They may be an antibacterial agent to de-stroy the acne-causing bacteria, a more powerful exfoliating agent to help shed the accumulated skin cells in the pore or follicle, and a drying agent to remove the excess sebum. Fighting inflamma-tion, which is part of every regimen, is especially important for people prone to breakouts, because the combination of bacteria, oil, and skin cells can trigger a destructive inflammatory response. This is an inclusive approach because it not only involves caring for your skin to accomplish all the wrinkle-fighting goals we've discussed, it also addresses each of the fac-tors causing your breakouts.

Environmentally Stressed or City Skin. If you live in an urban area, you are not only exposed to greater environmental toxins from pollution and smog, you also probably have a height-ened stress level that arises from just coping with the logistics of daily life. And if your city is in a very sunny part of the country, like Dallas, Miami, or Los Angeles, you also have a lot more daily sun exposure. In the city, busy work schedules often mean you rely on fast foods or high-fat restaurant meals and eat fewer fruits and vegetables. This kind of diet also contributes to skin problems.

Women who work in cities also tend to do more to their skin and it is often overprocessed. They wear more makeup, removing it and reapplying it sometimes twice a day, which can contribute to the irritation, too.

Also, despite the fact that cities are crowded, people work long hours and often live alone. I think this kind of isolation also contributes to skin problems.

Many of the steps in my program are designed to counter all these stresses. By flooding your skin with the materials it needs for optimal functioning, you're helping it defend itself against ultraviolet light and pollution as well as internal stress.

Sensitive Skin. People of all skin colors can have sensitive skin, but it is more common in those with a fair complexion and light-colored eyes. Your skin tends to sting when you put certain things on it, and you've probably learned over the years what to avoid. Your skin may even react to cold temperatures or wind by becoming red and irritated. You may also notice tiny cracks in your skin, and that makeup becomes flaky. In fact, the barrier function of skin in people with sensitivities has been disturbed, which is why it's so vulnerable to anything that's put on it.

Although the irritation—redness, stinging, itching, and burning—that you sometimes experience is not the same as a truly allergic reaction, you are more prone to true allergies, and you can break out in a rash all over if you are allergic to a fragrance or some other ingredient or drug.

With few exceptions, the formulations of my products are safe for most people with sensitive skin. Therefore I have not designed a separate daily regimen for this skin type. Usually, following the recommendations for dry skin will be fine for you. However, you may have an allergic response to some ingredient in any formulation, regardless of how much testing has been done to insure that it is unlikely to cause a reaction. So you might do your own skin test on the inside of your upper arm before using any product for the first time. Also, you can develop an allergy to something you have used without any problems for years, so don't ignore any unusual symptoms such as redness, rashes, irritation, stinging, or dry patches that occur when you use a product.

According to some surveys, about 40 percent of women say they have sensitive skin. They say their skin becomes red, itches, feels tight, stings, and burns in response to changes in the climate, in reaction to the sun, or when they use some products. No one knows how many people really have sensitive skin, but it is estimated that as many as 20 percent of people are allergic to certain things that make contact with their skin.

Menopausal Skin. Some dermatologists feel that the skin of people over forty should be treated differently. They say "mature skin" is a type in and of itself. I believe all adults have "mature" skin, and all of my products and the alternatives I suggest are for people of every age. However, women's skin is affected by the shifting balance of hormones just prior to, during, and after menopause.

Women who never had breakouts in their lives may find they now get pimples, as they have less estrogen to suppress the sebum-stimulating androgen circulating in their bodies. For the same reason, they may have more facial hair and they may perspire more. Also, because the skin thins so much with age, women past menopause may have more visible sun damage, such as brown spots and fine, dilated blood vessels, and increasingly sensitive skin. In fact, older women need to be even more watchful of the sun and weather extremes, such as cold and wind.

Although most physicians assume that only women have menopausal skin, I believe that men also have a shift in hormones in middle age. So men might find that the menopausal skin program works well for them.

SKIN DISEASES

There are far too many skin conditions to address individually in this book. Some of these problems, such as roseacea and folliculitis (inflammation of the hair follicle) are sometimes confused with acne. Others, such as psoriasis, initially appear as dry, flaky skin and may not be taken seriously until the condition is severe. If you have any kind of eruptions or severe or persistent skin problems, see a physician. You may need medical treatment in addition to following my advice for sensible skin care. Rarely, your dermatologist will find the care that I'm suggesting is contraindicated by his or her treatment. In general, the advice in this book is for those who do not have serious skin conditions.

However, if you have a skin condition you need to be aware that it does contribute to irritation and aging because they often create a break in the skin that disrupts the protective barrier function. Irritating substances and bacteria pass through this break and gain access to deeper layers of the skin as well as allow moisture to escape. You may still be able to follow my program, but you should discuss it with your physician first.

If you follow my program and make your skin as healthy as it can be, the barrier function will be intact, and all the skin layers will be protected and less susceptible to disrupting conditions. If problems do arise from some internal cause, skin that is already healthy, moist, and has all the building blocks it needs will be better able to cope with them.

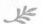

ELEVEN

How the Murad Program Works

All of the wrinkle fighters that you've just learned about should be incorporated into your daily skin care regimen. And everything you do—from cleansing to sun protection to special treatments—is an opportunity to flood your skin with anti-aging ingredients. My recipe, the basic ingredients needed to repair, maintain, and protect your skin, should be in everything you put on your skin. The daily supplements deliver the same wrinkle-fighting action to your skin from the inside.

My program for basic skin care includes four steps: cleansing, toning, treating and repairing, and moisturizing and protecting. Exfoliation, removing some of the dead skin cells from the stratum corneum that are no longer functioning, may be an aspect of both the cleansing and moisturizing steps, and it may be included in a treatment, depending on the products you use. Everyone over the age of twenty needs some type of exfoliation to counter the slowdown in cell turnover. How much exfoliation you need is unique to you. If you are using an exfoliating cleanser and moisturizer five days out of seven and your skin feels tight a half hour after you cleanse it, cut back to three days and then listen to your skin. If you exfoliate every other day and your skin is tolerating it well, try increasing it by one day and see how your skin responds.

SHOPPING FOR INGREDIENTS

I'll be recommending certain ingredients throughout this book that you may read elsewhere is irritating or drying. This causes a lot of confusion among consumers. What you may not realize is that one ingredient or another is not the only active compound in a product, and a good-quality product is a properly balanced mix that shouldn't cause problems for most people who use them. Of course, it's possible to have an allergy to an ingredient.

Cosmetic chemistry is a science, and product formulations are painstakingly developed so that the side effects of one ingredient are countered by the beneficial effects of others. Sometimes, too, one ingredient enhances the effectiveness of another. Each cosmetic company's formulation is unique, so while it is useful to shop for ingredients, keep in mind that the concentration and pH of products may vary, that different products use different "vehicles" in which the ingredients are mixed, and that it is the mix that matters. So ingredients, alone, are not the whole story.

As you will see as you look over the regimens that follow, there is not a single ingredient, product, or supplement that's suggested, but rather an orchestrated approach to skin care that includes all the wrinkle fighters described earlier. Just as your body needs a balance of proteins, fats, and carbohydrates, your skin needs a balance of hydrators, antioxidants, anti-inflammatory agents, collagen builders, and sun protectors. I call it an inclusive program because it really delivers the best of everything that your skin needs to be healthy.

HOLD ON TO THAT WATER

By now it should be permanently imprinted in your conscious-ness that your skin is a barrier, keeping harmful things out and helpful things—especially water—in. Every step of your skin care regimen is directed toward protecting that barrier and increasing your skin's water content.

You may think you know all there is to know about, say, wash-ing your face, but you may learn something new or clarify some misconception. Since you're going to be designing a prescription for yourself and modifying it as you try optional treatments and as your skin changes, be certain you know the basic principles. After all, you're investing time and money in following the program, so be sure you understand what you're doing and why.

Basic skin care may seem simple and straightforward, but I've found in talking with people that as knowledgeable as many of them are, they are susceptible to some misinformation. For instance, many people believe that the right product will shrink their enlarged pores. The truth is you can remove some of the debris that stretches the pores and makes them appear larger, but pore size is genetically determined and immutable.

The skin care regimens that follow are organized by skin type. You'll notice that all of them include similar hydrating ingredi-ents, antioxidants, skin soothers or anti-inflammatory agents, and collagen builders. In one step or another, though, there will be additional ingredients or variations on the recipe to address the needs of that particular skin type.

Everything that you do to meet your daily skin care needs should contain the appropriate ingredients. You want to cleanse your skin, treat it with anti-aging products, moisturize it, and pro-tect it with sunscreen. If you have special concerns, such as acne, you will need to make some modifications. You'll notice that I've provided regimens for those special concerns to make it easier for you. There are also optional suggestions within each skin type for some special needs or simply to suggest other products that you may want to use, such as eye cream.

Everyone can benefit from an extra antioxidant treatment each day, and most people can use an exfoliation boost, though the frequency and type can vary with skin type. As long as whatever you do is gentle, doesn't damage the skin's barrier function, and keeps water in the cells, you can't go wrong.

CLEANSE

Twice a day you need to wash your face to remove the dirt, debris, makeup, flakes of dead skin cells, and accumulated oils. And you want to remove all this surface material without disturbing your skin's barrier function. A good cleanser and warm—not hot—water will gently do this. It will dissolve the material on the skin's surface and allow it to be rinsed away without injuring that vital barrier.

No matter how gentle a cleanser you use, removing some of the structural lipids from the stratum corneum is unavoidable. Just splashing your face with water will remove some of these lipids.

Knowing this, I wonder why people with dry skin think that if they just splash their face with water, they don't need to worry about moisturizing. Also overcleansing—that is, washing your face several times a day—can lead to dryness. With the appropriate cleanser followed immediately by a moisturizer, most people can tolerate at least twice-a-day cleansing. You will be able to tell if you are overdoing it. For example, if your skin feels "squeaky-clean" or tight, the cleanser you're using is not gentle enough. Sometimes, I suggest that people with very dry and/or sensitive skin try using a moisture-rich cleanser that is tissued off and avoid water entirely.

Men don't usually have such dry skin. Women are more likely to be troubled with dryness because they have fewer pores and oil glands and their skin is so dramatically affected by hormones—or a lack of them.

Aggressive cleansing doesn't benefit any skin type, including oily skin. That is because when the protective shield of the epidermis is disrupted, the skin becomes more vulnerable to environmental damage and inflammation, and precious moisture escapes. I have found that when a person with oily skin uses an appropriate cleanser, there is no harm in cleansing three times a day. And no one, regardless of skin type, should use a cleanser that leaves a greasy film on the skin. It may give the barrier function a little boost, but it also attracts impurities and clogs the pores, so the disadvantages outweigh the benefits.

Gentle cleansing products are water soluble, which is just another way of saying the cleanser dissolves in water, which most of them do. Oils and fatty acids such as stearic acid and glycerol stearate may be added to some cleansers to help hold the ingredients together. There are also detergents, such as sodium lauryl sulfate, that also assist in removing oils. Whether or not these ingredients will irritate the skin depends on how much of them is in the cleanser.

Few ingredients are actually harmful, but the formulation may not be right for your skin. So choosing a cleanser is a bit of a trial-and-error process. Even when I see patients in my office and have the opportunity to directly examine their skin, I may prescribe a cleanser that is too drying or not drying enough, and we have to try another one. I always ask patients to try to be aware of how their skin feels a half hour after they wash their face when they don't use a moisturizer right away. If it feels dry, taut, and stiff, the cleanser is too harsh and another one must be tried.

What you want is skin that feels soft and pliable a half hour after you wash your face. I feel very strongly that you have to take the frequently heard advice to "listen to your body" and apply it to your skin. You will know if your skin is responding well to how you're treating it. Everyone has a certain level of tolerance, a comfort zone. Know what your skin can handle and respect its limits.

There are some cleansing ingredients that I have found to be very useful for certain skin types. For example, an ingredient that disperses oil called farnesol is sometimes used in cleansers for oily skin. Instead of stripping the skin of oil, as most cleansers for this skin type tend to do, the farnesol disperses the oil. You feel less oily, and not too many of the structural lipids that keep the water balance have been removed. The skin's barrier is intact.

A cleanser with hydroxy acids, such as glycolic and salicylic acids, is useful for most people because they exfoliate the skin during cleansing and enhance hydration. Depending on your skin type, you may want to use an AHA/BHA skin cleanser every day, once a week, or two or three times a week. A gentle hydroxy acid–containing cleanser should also contain anti-irritant ingredients such as allantoin or the emollient B vitamin panthenol. Panthenol is so helpful that Europeans often use it to treat diaper rash.

Some people argue that putting active ingredients like hydroxy acids or vitamins in cleansers is a waste of money, since the cleanser is rinsed away in a few minutes. Active ingredients do add to the cost of a product, but I believe that when the formulation is effective, these ingredients do penetrate the top layers of the skin as you massage the cleanser over your face.

If you have troubled skin and you are at risk for developing infections, you may benefit from infection fighters like triclosan, which have long been used in deodorants and soaps. Triclosan can clear nearly all of the bacteria on the skin's surface in less than a minute. This helps to prevent infection that can arise when people pick at their pimples. Triclosan does not, however, penetrate deeply into the pores to kill the bacteria that contributes to acne, so remember as you read labels that "antiseptic" doesn't always mean "acne fighter."

Women who wear makeup sometimes use a cleansing cream or makeup remover before they wash their faces. I don't think this is necessary, unless you use a very greasy or waterproof makeup. A water-soluble cleanser and warm water will remove most types of foundation. The fewer things you use on your skin the better, and in most cases there's no reason to use two cleansers.

If you must use a makeup remover, then apply it only where you need it. For instance, if you have black circles under your eyes from your mascara, then use an eye-makeup remover on the skin beneath the eyes.

Many people believe that tugging on their skin can cause wrinkles, and so they always use an upward and/or circular motion when cleansing. I'm not sure where the idea that massage, even quite vigorous massage, causes wrinkles comes from, but of all the things that contribute to aging skin, rubbing or pulling or massaging it aren't anywhere near the top of the list. Of course, you don't want to be too rough with your skin, because rubbing very hard with an abrasive scrub, sponge, or loofah can be irritating. But much of the advice people have heard about hands-on cleansing has no basis in fact.

There are many, many cleansers that remove dirt and debris gently and easily. You could keep it simple and choose a cleanser that only does that. However, my philosophy is that everything you do for or to your skin should also replenish it with wrinkle fighters. That is why I suggest looking for a cleanser that includes a hydrator, such as sodium PCA, or a lipid, such as hyaluronic acid, to help restore some of the skin's own natural structural lipids that are lost every time you put water on your face. I also encourage people to take advantage of every opportunity to reduce irritation and inflammation, which are such important factors in aging. For this reason, I recommend cleansers that are

Q & A

I'm thirty-five and work in the fashion industry, which requires me to wear more makeup than I would like. Every day I wear foundation and powder, concealer around my eyes, and eye shadow, mascara, and blush. The first thing I want to do when I get home is wash it all off, so on most weekdays I'm washing my face three times a day. My pores are fine and I tend to have dry skin. What should I use to take off my makeup? Am I washing my face too much? What can I do to avoid drying it even further?

First of all, you don't need to wash your face three times a day. Remove your makeup with a cleansing cream or makeup remover when you get home and then let it be. The more you wash, the more dry and irritated your skin will be. At bedtime use a gentle cleanser, your exfoliating and hydrating treatment, and apply a night cream. The next morning, follow your cleansing and vitamin C treatment with a moisturizer. On the weekends, when you don't need to wear as much makeup, if any, give your skin a break and cleanse just once a day, if you can. You don't have to do the same thing every day. Dry skin can use a rest from cleansing occasionally.

infused with anti-irritant agents like licorice extract or chamomile. Vitamin E also is an excellent skin soother.

TONE

Toners are often promoted for restoring the skin's pH or its "acid mantle." It's true that skin functions best when its pH is about 4.5 to 5.5, or slightly acid, and most gentle cleansers have a slightly alkaline pH of about 8. (Normal pH—that is, neither acid nor alkaline—is 7). A toner, with a pH of 3 to 7, will encourage the skin to return to a slightly acid pH.

The reality is that the skin will rapidly restore the pH to about 5 on its own. A toner may accomplish it within seconds, but the few minutes' difference is inconsequential in terms of skin health. (In some cases a treatment product, such as my Essential C Daily Renewal Complex, requires moisture for activation, and some people use a spray of toner instead of water.)

For those who like to use a toner, I have two recommendations. First, look for one that doesn't contain an irritating, drying type of alcohol. (Not all alcohol is drying, and some types are actually hydrating, so again, "listen to your skin.") Witch hazel is often used, and I don't find that it's irritating for most people. If you have sensitive skin, use a fragrance-free toner. It's often the fixatives that are used with fragrance that cause reactions, so products with only essential oils for scent may be tolerated by those with sensitive skin. Second, as with cleansers, a toner is another opportunity to supply your skin with active ingredients to help maintain the barrier function of the skin.

There are skin-soothing botanicals in some toners, such as mint, coneflower, chamomile, and/or bitter orange. Any ingredi-

Q & A

My skin is very oily. To avoid a slick look, I have to wash my face after lunch at the office and reapply makeup. I usually use a mild cleanser and those little disposable abrasive sponges. Someone told me that I'm only irritating my skin with all this scrubbing and actually increasing the activity of my oil glands. Is this true? I like the "clean" feeling that I get after using the sponges, but I'm wondering if I'm making my oily skin even worse.

Hormones and other internal agents control oil production from the sebaceous glands, not massage, face washing, or anything else you do to care for your skin. Instead of washing your face so often, though, try using rice paper to blot the oil. You press the paper to your skin, on top of your makeup, and it quickly absorbs the excess oil. You might do this two or three times a day. You won't have to spend the time reapplying your makeup and you'll avoid irritating your skin with so much washing.

ent that helps reduce irritation will also diminish aging free radicals. Also, some toners contain hydrating ingredients like sodium PCA and/or amino acids that enhance hydration. And, of course, antioxidants, such as vitamins C and E, help disarm free radicals.

People with oily skin who rely on toners that use a drying

type of alcohol need to be careful not to overuse them. I suggest they use this type of toner no more than twice a day. The reason for this caution is that stripping oil from the skin's surface also removes the moisture-holding lipids that are needed to keep the skin hydrated. Using a toner with natural moisture factors, such as sodium PCA, can also counteract this effect.

TREAT AND REPAIR

Every step of your daily regimen is important, but the most powerful anti-aging step is treat and repair. While cleansing, toning, moisturizing, and protecting products include my anti-aging

Q & A

I have combination oily-dry skin, and I tend to break out on the sides of my nose. Should I use a drying alcohol toner on those oily areas or will that dry out my skin too much?

For breakouts anywhere on the skin I recommend an acne spot treatment product. However, if breakouts occur on a weekly basis, you might use an all-over acne treatment that is less potent than the spot treatment as a preventive. Remember, since oil is not the cause of acne, using a drying alcohol toner may not be beneficial.

recipe, they each have another purpose in addition to fighting wrinkles. Their formulations include ingredients to remove surface debris, for instance, or protect against ultraviolet light.

In contrast, the recommendations I make in the treat-and-repair category are designed to repair any damage that's already been done and optimize the health of your skin so it can defend itself against further injury. For example, every day, regardless of your skin type, you will have at least one internal and external antioxidant treatment that contains mostly vitamin C. This portion of the program also includes the supplements that will accomplish your internal skin care regimen, feeding your skin the same basic anti-aging recipe from the inside.

I think of the products I suggest for treatment and repair as the booster shots of your regimen. The supplements are treating and repairing your skin from the inside, and the skin care products are doing the same from the outside. At least twice a day—in the morning and at night—you'll be giving yourself at least one internal and one external booster treatment. The vitamin C treatment is always recommended in the morning, because you're flooding your skin with antioxidants that can combat the day's environmental abuse. The vitamin C is hydrating as well. Typically, the evening treatment is predominately an exfoliating and hydrating treatment, but it also contains an antioxidant. You'll take your collagen builder and antioxidant supplements in the morning and at night.

In the "Optional" column of some of the regimens, I've made other suggestions that you can use in addition to or alternate with those in the "Treat and Repair" column. And some, such as the Acne Spot Treatment, are to be used only as needed. What you use from the optional column and how often you use it depends entirely on your individual needs.

You have learned how vitamin C fights free radicals and inflammation and helps rebuild collagen. Many of the products you use, from cleansers to sunscreen, contain vitamin C, but to keep your skin richly supplied with this potent antioxidant, I suggest a daily treatment that contains over 10 percent ascorbic acid. Then, at least once a week, I recommend a supplemental infusion treatment with a 30 percent concentration of vitamin C. For maximum wrinkle fighting, you can have a professional facial by an esthetician or physician who uses an even higher, 40 percent concentration of vitamin C. These recommendations are based on the formulas I've designed. When you go shopping for a vitamin C treatment product, you probably won't find the percentage on the label. However, most vitamin C treatment products are about 10 to 15 percent formulations.

Most skin types can also benefit from the daily use of a hydroxy acid treatment. Even if the cleanser and moisturizer you use contain one or more hydroxy acids, a daily booster treatment of hydroxy acid will accelerate the exfoliation process. As a result, you will enhance hydration, smooth the skin, and increase cell turnover.

Depending on your skin type and the other steps in your regimen, you may want to use a topical product that boosts collagen, such as retinol or retinyl palmitate.

HYDRATE

Applying a moisturizer after every cleansing will immediately replenish the skin with structural lipids, smooth the rough, dry surface cells, and seal the barrier of the stratum corneum. A good moisturizer contains a mix of water-attracting and water-holding ingredients. Keep in mind, though, that as with every other product, it's the total formulation that affects how the moisturizer feels on your skin as well as its hydrating potential. For example, two moisturizers can contain similar ingredients, yet one will be more *occlusive* than the other, making it better for dry skin that needs that kind of invisible, nongreasy, water-holding shield. One moisturizer may work better under a foundation. And some women prefer a tinted moisturizer with sunscreen when they're not wearing a foundation. Men may prefer a moisturizer with more soothing ingredients to use after shaving.

Although most moisturizers are meant to be slightly occlusive, many of those on the market today don't make the skin feel greasy. In the past, petrolatum or mineral oil was often used in a moisturizer because of its occlusive properties. With the new technology available to cosmetic chemists, though, these sticky products have been replaced with lightweight ones that are even more effective. They often contain ceramides that seem to dissolve right into your skin. Ceramides boost hydration and immediately impart a silky texture to the skin.

In the past most moisturizers were available in either a water-in-oil formulation or an oil-in-water one. People with dry skin were encouraged to use the water-in-oil products that were more occlusive; and people who produced too much sebum or structural lipids were advised to use oil-in-water products. These distinctions are now outdated, as new ingredients and manufacturing processes have improved the formulations.

New delivery systems are also now incorporated into many moisturizers. The liposome, for instance, involves a kind of encapsulation process that transports whatever agent is put within the liposome into the epidermis. In contrast, biovectors can be attached to ingredients to keep them at the top of the skin. For instance, I use a biovector in some moisturizer formulas to hold the antioxidant grape seed extract in the stratum corneum, where it can boost the barrier defenses of this topmost skin layer.

WHY NIGHT CREAMS?

A night cream is a moisturizer in which there is a greater concentration of hydrating ingredients than is typically used in a day cream or lotion. Because of this richness, night creams may leave the skin with a slight occlusive layer that many people would not be comfortable wearing during the day or under foundation.

There are two reasons why a night cream is useful. One is that transepidermal water loss (TEWL) is greatest at night, and a night cream can help prevent that kind of dehydration. Two is that the body's cells are replenished with nutrients and are being regenerated at night, so this is the time to optimize the delivery of the raw materials skin needs. Now, too, is when free radical damage from the environment is at its lowest point. You're indoors, in the dark, and not active, so fewer free radicals are being produced within your skin as well. You can take advantage of this break in the action to disarm the free radicals that have accumulated during the day and saturate the skin with an extra supply so that you don't start the next day unprotected.

My patients often ask whether they should use a cream or a lotion. You may have heard that a cream has more oil than water or that a lotion has more water than oil. This is not completely accurate. Regardless of the oil-water balance, thickening agents give a product the consistency of a cream, not the oil.

WHY EYE CREAMS ARE DIFFERENT

The skin around the eyes is thin and absorbs moisturizing ingredients more rapidly than skin on other areas of the face. Because it is so delicate, it is also susceptible to irritation. There are no sebaceous glands in the eye area either, so there is less natural lubrication. Eye creams are formulated with all these differences in mind. They usually contain the same ingredients as moisturizers used on the face, but in a more gentle formula than products used on other areas.

The tissues around the eye are so delicate and prone to so many different age-related problems that most eye creams also deliver ingredients to do more than hydrate the skin. For instance, I think a good eye cream should contain caffeine to reduce the amount of water in the spaces between the cells that cause puffiness, vitamin K to help constrict dilated blood vessels, vitamin C to prevent damage from free radicals, skin soothers to reduce inflammation, and wrinkle fighters such as retinol. A nonirritating sunscreen in the cream protects this thin skin from ultraviolet radiation. And, finally, it may contain ingredients that reflect light to help minimize the appearance of dark circles and under-eye bags. So you see that an eye cream can be far more than a souped-up moisturizer.

I have noticed that some women misuse eye creams. They think the cream should be used over the upper lid and beneath the eye, up to the lower lashes. These areas are especially sensitive to irritation. And since the skin is so thin, any cream applied above and below the lid eventually will be absorbed further up. So it's safest, and just as helpful, to apply eye creams around the eye along the edge of the bone that outlines the eye socket.

Typically women prefer creamier moisturizers, and men prefer lotions that don't have thickening agents. But a lotion can be just as hydrating as a cream. In fact, one of the most popular moisturizing products in my line is neither a lotion nor a cream, but a viscous liquid. It's a combination of only water-attracting natural moisture factors and water-holding lipids. It's light and is absorbed immediately into the skin, moistening and smoothing the stratum corneum and leaving no trace on the skin's surface.

I believe that everyone, even those people with oily skin, needs to use a moisturizer. The idea of a moisturizer is not to add structural lipids alone. Rather, a moisturizer serves several purposes: smoothing, hydrating, and restoring the barrier function of the stratum corneum.

PROTECT

Despite all the public service announcements, magazine articles, and news stories, people continue to burn and tan. A study of over thirty thousand Americans who completed a National Health Interview Survey found that adult men and women were less likely than they were six years earlier to wear protective clothing, seek shade when outdoors, or wear sunscreen. Only about a third of those surveyed used sunscreen regularly.

As a dermatologist who sees the ravages of photodamage all

day nearly every day, I can tell you that nothing will give you youthful-looking skin if you continue to let yourself be bombarded with ultraviolet radiation. Using a sunscreen every day and taking a pomegranate supplement to boost its power are the critical protective steps of your daily regimen.

Many people prefer an all-occasion sunscreen that they wear every day regardless of their activities or the weather. Others have a range of products to use depending on what they're doing. A woman might use a sunscreen-boosted foundation or tinted moisturizer that contains titanium dioxide every workday, and then switch to a higher SPF sunscreen on weekends when she's spending more time outdoors gardening or playing golf. A man might use an SPF 15 moisturizer after shaving every morning and an

Q & A

I'm very fair and burn easily. Now that so many products have sunscreen in them, I'm able to use an SPF 15 moisturizer and an SPF 15 foundation. Am I getting the equivalent of SPF 30 protection?

Not really, though you are further insuring that the coverage you are getting is that of an SPF 15 sunscreen. It's like putting two coats of paint on a wall to get better coverage. Also, most people don't apply sunscreen liberally enough, and by using an SPF 15 moisturizer and an SPF 15 foundation, you're sure to be using enough.

SPF 30+, broad-spectrum, water-resistant product when he's playing tennis. Think of buying sun protection products as you would clothing. You have different shoes and coats for different occasions, why not a wardrobe of sun protection?

Q & A

I can buy a very large container of sunscreen at the discount store for a fraction of the cost of a department store or salon brand. The labels on both say "broad spectrum, SPF 30+." Is there any difference in their effectiveness?

Probably not, in terms of the amount of sun protection ingredients in the products. But there are other qualities that make a difference, and so there may be other ingredients in one sunscreen but not in another. For instance, is the inexpensive sunscreen also water-resistant? Does it have a pleasant scent? Does it absorb into your skin nicely? If a product smells awful or doesn't go on smoothly, you're less likely to use it as often as you need to. Now look at the list of ingredients. Does it contain an antioxidant? An anti-inflammatory? A moisturizer? These ingredients do increase the cost of a product, but by using them you are also curtailing other harmful effects of sun exposure, such as inflammation, free radicals, and dehydration.

To get the full sun-screening protection from whatever product you use, you have to apply it early, liberally, and often. Ideally, you need to apply your sunscreen on a half hour before you go outside, again a half hour after being outside, and then every two hours that you remain in the sun. If you perspire heavily or you are swimming, you need to reapply sunscreen more often. And use at least an ounce to cover your entire body. If you use less, you aren't getting the same SPF protection that's stated on the product label.

SPECIAL CONCERNS

There are certain conditions that require special attention, and while some are more often linked to a particular skin type—like acne and oily skin—they can occur in anyone. It's unusual, but I occasionally see an older person with dry skin who is troubled by breakouts. For those with special concerns, there are regimens that include different treat-and-repair steps. The special concerns that I see most often are hyperpigmentation, acne, environmentally stressed skin, which I call "city skin," and menopausal skin.

TWELVE

The Murad Program

You'll find a Murad Program that suits your skin's specific needs on the following pages. The programs include all the wrinkle fighters in my anti-aging recipe, and they are categorized broadly by skin type. In the "Optional" column you will find some suggested products that you may want to use in addition to your basic treat-and-repair step on a daily or occasional basis, depending on what your skin requires. And don't forget the supplements. This is as important a step in the program as the products you see in the treat-and-repair step.

A "Special Concerns" section follows the daily regimens. If you are troubled with a special concern that is not addressed in your skin type, you can alternate the recommended treat-and-repair step in the Special Concerns chart for that step in your skin type program. Or, if your special concern is severe, you can substitute the recommendations given in this chart for those in your skin type program.

In the Murad Program, I recommend my own formulations, because I've personally designed and tested them and know they work. If you choose to use products other than mine, go to the appendix and find suggested alternatives for your skin type. As I've said throughout this book, formulations do vary and products may contain the same ingredients but in different amounts and combinations. This is where you'll have to do some experimenting and listen to your skin. If a product is too harsh for you, or you're not seeing the desired result after five weeks, try another formulation. In the appendix is a listing of products and their main ingredients, so if you choose to customize your own program, the job will be less daunting.

NORMAL/COMBINATION

My anti-aging recipe will make good skin even better by creating the best internal environment for skin cells to perform at their optimal level. The healthier your skin is, the better able it is to cope with the challenges of time, sun, and stress. Think of the plants in your home. You not only water them to keep them healthy, you also give them plant food, spray them with water, reposition them when the light changes, remove the dead leaves, and maybe even pinch back the old growth so that the new growth is more strong and healthy. Normal skin is like that, too. You not only keep it clean and hydrated, you nourish it and do what you can to make it even more resilient.

In the morning, use a cleanser that is rich in skin soothers, followed with a hydrating toner. Then, while the skin is still moist, give it a boost of antioxidants to combat the free radicals in the environment. Give the antioxidant treatment a few minutes to seep into your skin, then seal in all those powerful free-radical fighters with a light, vitamin-enriched moisturizer. For sun protection, you'll want to use an oil-free sunblock.

In the morning take your multivitamin; calcium; and fatty

acid, antioxidant, and collagen-building supplements. To boost the power of your sunblock, take a pomegranate supplement as well.

In the evening, after cleansing and toning, treat your skin with an exfoliating product, and follow it with the same moisturizer you used in the morning.

In the evening, take fatty acid and antioxidant and collagen-building supplements.

You may want to vary your regimen with a bit more exfoliation if your skin can tolerate it. I often suggest alternating the usual cleanser with one that contains hydroxy acids three or more times a week. Also, if your skin can tolerate it, use a higher concentration of hydroxy acids for your evening treatment (see the "Optional" column).

Every week, give yourself a special vitamin C treatment to saturate your skin with a high concentration of antioxidants. And if you can, have a professional vitamin C infusion at least once a season.

NORMAL/COMBINATION SKIN

	Cleanse	Tone	Treat and Repair	Hydrate	Protect	Optional
MORNING	Murad Refreshing Cleanser	Murad Hydrating Toner	Murad Essential-C Daily Renewal Complex -Internal- Murad Pomphenol Sunguard Supplement Murad Youth Builder Collagen Supplement Murad Daily Renewal Complex Antioxidant Supplement Murad Wet Suit Hydrating Supplement Coenzyme Q 10	Murad Skin Perfecting Lotion	Murad Oil-Free Sunblock SPF 15	Murad Waterproof Sunblock SPF 30 Murad Essential-C Eye Cream SPF 15
EVENING	Murad Refreshing Cleanser	Murad Hydrating Toner	Murad Combination Skin Treatment	Murad Skin Perfecting Lotion		Murad Acne Spot Treatment

	Cleanse	Tone	Treat and Repair	Hydrate	Protect	Optional
			-Internal- Murad Daily Renewal Complex Antioxidant Supplement Murad Youth Builder Collagen Supplement Murad Wet Suit Hydrating Supplement Coenzyme Q 10			Murad Night Reform Treatment Murad Eye Treatment Complex SPF 8
WEEKLY OR MORE	Murad AHA/BHA Exfoliating Cleanser					
WEEKLY			Murad Vitamin C Infusion System			

OILY SKIN

Oily skin isn't unhealthy. The oil glands within the follicles are simply genetically programmed to be more active in response to hormonal stimulation. This stepped-up production of sebum is bothersome because the oil gives skin a shiny appearance. Although oily skin is perceived as being moist, it may actually lack sufficient structural lipids. So one of the main objectives of this regimen is to reduce the shine without removing too much of the skin's natural moisturizers, which help optimize the skin's water content.

I recommend a cleanser that is a little more active in removing the surface oils than the one I suggest for normal/combination skin. The toner is similar. You may want to work more exfoliation into your regimen by using a cleanser with hydroxy acids on alternate days or more often if your skin seems to respond well to it.

Then, while the skin is still moist from the toner, give it a boost of antioxidants to combat the free radicals in the environment. Allow the antioxidant treatment a few minutes to seep into your skin, then seal in all those powerful free radical–fighting ingredients with a light, vitamin-enriched moisturizer. For sun protection, use an oil-free sunblock. The micronized particles of titanium give your skin a matte finish that helps minimize the shine of oily skin.

In the morning you'll take your multivitamin, calcium, fatty acids, and antioxidant and collagen-building supplements. To boost the power of your sunblock, take a pomegranate supplement as well.

In the evening, you'll treat your skin to an overall acne treatment product that not only addresses the various factors that contribute to breakouts but contains collagen builders, such as retinol, along with exfoliating and hydrating ingredients. If you do have an occasional breakout, you can apply a more potent acne

OILY SKIN

	Cleanse	Tone	Treat and Repair	Hydrate	Protect	Optional
MORNING	Murad Clarifying Cleanser	Murad Clarifying Toner	Murad Essential-C Daily Renewal Complex -Internal- Murad Pomphenol Sunguard Supplement Murad Youth Builder Collagen Supplement Murad Daily Renewal Complex Antioxidant Supplement Murad Wet Suit Hydrating Supplement Coenzyme Q 10	Murad Skin Perfecting Lotion	Murad Oil-Free Sunblock SPF 15 Sheer Tint	Murad Waterproof Sunblock SPF 30 Murad Essential-C Eye Cream SPF 15

OILY SKIN

	Cleanse	Tone	Treat and Repair	Hydrate	Protect	Optional
EVENING	Murad Clarifying Cleanser	Murad Clarifying Toner	Murad Moisturizing Acne Treatment Gel -Internal- Murad Youth Builder Collagen Supplement Murad Daily Renewal Complex Antioxidant Supplement Murad Wet Suit Hydrating Supplement Coenzyme Q 10	Murad Cellular Replenishing Serum		Murad Night Reform Treatment Murad Eye Treatment Complex SPF 8

	Cleanse	Tone	Treat and Repair	Hydrate	Protect	Optional
WEEKLY OR MORE	Murad AHA/BHA Exfoliating Cleanser					
WEEKLY			Murad Vitamin C Infusion System			

spot treatment. However, if breakouts are a daily problem, see "Acne" in the Special Concerns Program.

You can follow the treat-and-repair step with a moisturizer of structural lipids and soothing botanicals only. You don't need an emollient or occlusive moisturizer at night.

In the evening, take fatty acids and antioxidant and collagen-building supplements.

Every week, you'll give yourself a special vitamin C treatment to saturate your skin with antioxidants. And if you can, have a professional vitamin C infusion at least once every season.

DRY SKIN

Your skin is the most fragile of all the skin types. The lack of oil and structural lipids allows the moisture to escape into the environment. And the dryness and the compromised barrier function have made your skin vulnerable to irritants and inflammation. The emphasis of every step in every regimen is hydration, but delivering water-attracting and water-holding molecules to the skin is especially important to you. Avoiding anything that might irritate is crucial. In some cases where some mild irritation is unavoidable—such as with exfoliation—you need even more skin soothers in everything you use.

Your cleanser must be very gentle, and I suggest one that has more hydrating ingredients than anything else. If your skin is very dry, I suggest that for at least one of the two times a day that you cleanse your face, you don't rinse with water but tissue off the cleanser.

The toner you choose should not contain a drying type of alcohol but must be rich in hydrating and skin-soothing ingredients.

Then, while the skin is still moist from the toner, give it a boost of antioxidants to combat the free radicals in the environment. Give the antioxidant treatment a few minutes to seep into your skin, and then seal in all those powerful free radical–fighting ingredients with a light, vitamin-enriched moisturizer.

If you need extra sun protection, choose a sunscreen with chemicals that absorb light as well as micronized titanium to block ultraviolet radiation. You also want your sunscreen to contain soothing botanicals and structural lipids. An oil-free sunblock may be too drying for your skin.

If your skin begins to feel dry and tight during the day, try a moisturizing serum that is primarily structural lipids. You can use one that contains only structural lipids or one that also includes skin-soothing botanical extracts. Or you can use both and alternate between them.

In the morning you'll take your multivitamin, calcium, fatty acids, and antioxidant and collagen-building supplements. To boost the power of your sunblock, take a pomegranate supplement as well.

In the evening, after cleansing and toning, you'll treat your skin with an exfoliating product that also contains the least irritating collagen builder, retinyl palmitate. Follow the treat-and-repair step with a very emollient moisturizer.

In the evening, take fatty acids and antioxidant and collagen-building supplements.

You may want to vary your program with a bit more exfoliation if your skin can tolerate it. I often suggest alternating the usual cleanser with one that contains hydroxy acids every two or three days. Also, you may want to use a higher concentration of hydroxy acids for your evening treatment. (See the "Optional" column).

Every week, give yourself a special vitamin C infusion treatment to saturate your skin with antioxidants. And if you can, have a professional vitamin C infusion at least once every season.

DRY SKIN

	Cleanse	Tone	Treat and Repair	Hydrate	Protect	Optional
MORNING	Murad Moisture Rich Cleanser	Murad Hydrating Toner	Murad Essential-C Daily Renewal Complex -Internal- Murad Pomphenol Sunguard Supplement Murad Youth Builder Collagen Supplement Murad Daily Renewal Complex Antioxidant Supplement Murad Wet Suit Hydrating Supplement Coenzyme Q 10	Murad Perfecting Day Cream SPF 15	Murad Hydrating Sunscreen SPF 15	Murad Waterproof Sunblock SPF 30 Murad Essential-C Eye Cream SPF 15 Murad Perfecting Serum
EVENING	Murad Moisture Rich Cleanser	Murad Hydrating Toner	Murad Skin Smoothing Treatment	Murad Perfecting Night Cream		Murad Night Reform Treatment

	Cleanse	Tone	Treat and Repair	Hydrate	Protect	Optional
			Internal- Murad Youth Builder Collagen Supplement Murad Daily Renewal Complex Antioxidant Supplement Murad Wet Suit Hydrating Supplement Coenzyme Q 10			Murad Eye Treatment Complex SPF 8 Murad Perfecting Serum
WEEKLY	Murad AHA/BHA Exfoliating Cleanser		Murad Vitamin C Infusion System			

SPECIAL CONCERNS

It's not unusual to have an occasional bout of breakouts or to have mildly hyperpigmented areas on our faces, and most of us are exposed to pollution or overtreat our skin from time to time, but when these situations are extreme, treating them consistently needs to become part of your daily program. The recommendations I make to remedy these problems can be used as needed. In some cases, you may have to shift your priorities, changing your program entirely to deal with a particular skin problem. Then, when it's under control, you can go back to the wrinkle-fighting program for your skin type.

You'll see on page 172 a chart of treat-and-repair recommendations for each special concern. You can use this in addition to the treat-and-repair program provided for your skin type, or you can alternate the program for your skin type on one day with the program for your special concern on the next day. As with all the recommendations I make, listen to your skin when treating a special concern. If you have acne, for instance, and your skin can tolerate the acne program every day, then use it instead of the program for your skin type. However, if using the evening Murad Exfoliating Acne Treatment Gel is too irritating for you—and it may be if you have, say, dry skin—then use it every other day, or every two days until your acne clears.

Hyperpigmentation. The most common treatment for too much pigment or uneven distribution of melanin, known as hyperpigmentation, is hydroquinone. It's not exactly bleach, though some people refer to products that contain hydroquinone as skin-bleaching creams. Hydroquinone lightens the skin by inhibiting the chemical reactions that create melanin. It can be combined with an alpha hydroxy acid, such as glycolic acid,

which increases cell turnover. The skin cells with the extra pigment are shed more quickly, and pigmentation in the new skin
cells is more uniform.

Over-the-counter skin lighteners that contain a 2 percent
concentration of hydroquinone or less are adequate for most people. Higher concentrations are available by prescription. There are
also prescription formulations that combine hydroquinone with
Retin-A and other ingredients. I don't usually recommend these
prescription products because I think that while they have some
immediate benefits, in the long run they're too irritating and may
actually contribute to pigment problems. I often suggest that people alternate hydroquinone-containing products with those that
contain other types of brightening agents, or use one type of
lightener in the morning, the other at night.

Pregnant or nursing women should not use hydroquinone,
because the appropriate safety studies have never been done.

City Skin. For most urban dwellers, taking themselves to the
country to decompress every few days isn't an option, so I suggest
using the vitamin C treatment twice a day. For exfoliation, I recommend alternating an evening treatment that contains hydroxy
acids with the vitamin C treatment.

Menopausal Skin. There are ingredients that cause facial hair
to thin and slow its growth, so that women who wax areas of their
faces, which is quite irritating, don't have to do it so often.

Women who never had breakouts in their lives may find they
now get pimples and they may need to use an acne spot treatment
from time to time. Also, because the skin thins so much with age,
if you are a woman past menopause you may have more visible
sun damage, such as brown spots and fine, dilated blood vessels.
You not only need to use a lightening product and topical vitamin
C for the brown spots, you also need anti-inflammatory agents to

soothe your increasingly sensitive skin. In fact, older women need to be even more watchful of the sun and weather extremes, such as cold and wind. You may need more skin-soothing ingredients in the products you use. Skin cell turnover in menopausal skin is even more sluggish, so a gentle exfoliating treatment every evening is essential.

I've also formulated a night cream, Age-Balancing Night Cream, with extra hydrating botanical oils, retinol, a hair-growth inhibitor, and a firming ingredient.

Although the tendency is to assume that only women have menopausal skin, I believe that men also have a shift in hormones as they become senior citizens. So middle-aged men might find that the menopausal skin program works well for them, too.

Acne. The most effective acne treatment products contain a cocktail of ingredients that work on different aspects of the conditions. For instance, alpha hydroxy acids help eliminate the dead skin cells that block the pore. The beta hydroxy acid, salicylic acid, assists skin cell removal, too, as well as promotes healing. Depending on your skin type, you may want to use a cleanser with hydroxy acids at least once a day.

In addition to the morning vitamin C treatment, which will combat the free radicals that result from the inflammation of acne as well as those created by environmental factors, you need a treatment product that contains antiseptic ingredients to rid the skin of superficial bacteria. Since your skin is likely to be inflamed and irritated, you also need zinc and soothing allantoin. Many of these can be combined in one product that delivers vitamins A and C, zinc, and skin-soothing botanicals.

If your acne fails to respond to this program and a daily anti-acne supplement, see a physician. You may need a prescription for internal and/or topical antibiotics to break the acne cycle where it starts deep within the pore or follicle. For some women birth control pills or estrogen replacement therapy may correct the hormonal imbalance. And, of course, learning how to minimize the stress in your life can help clear your skin.

In the case of serious acne that doesn't respond to standard treatments, Accutane, a form of vitamin A, may be prescribed. This drug is quite effective in acne treatment, but there are side effects, such as extreme dryness. This is a good example of how a drug can alter your skin type. Women who take Accutane must take precautions to prevent pregnancy and have periodic pregnancy tests. Both men and women need frequent blood tests to monitor their health.

For sun protection, use an oil-free sunblock. The micronized particles of titanium give your skin a matte finish that helps minimize the shine of oily skin.

In the morning you'll take your multivitamin; calcium; essential fatty acids; and antioxidant, collagen-building, and anti-acne supplements. To boost the power of your sunblock, take a pomegranate supplement as well.

In the evening, you'll use the same acne treatment product and follow with a lightweight moisturizer. If necessary, you can apply a more potent spot treatment to any active lesions. Also at night, you'll repeat your regimen of supplements.

Sensitive Skin. This regimen is very similar to that used for the person with dry skin, with more emphasis on hydration and skin soothing to reduce inflammation. The barrier function of sensitive skin is typically very compromised, so the moisturizing ingredients are essential to help restore that barrier. I suggest doing a little patch test on any new product you use on your skin, even if the label says it's for sensitive skin. This is very easy to do—just rub a dot of the product on the inside of your upper arm and check it the next day. If there is any redness signaling irritation, don't use the product.

TREAT AND REPAIR SPECIAL CONCERNS

	Hyperpigmentation	City Skin (overprocessed)	Menopausal	Acne	Sensitive
MORNING	Murad Brightening Treatment SPF 15 (Alternate)	Murad Essential-C Daily Renewal Complex -Internal- Murad Vital Spark Supplement	Murad Essential-C Daily Renewal Complex	Murad Essential-C Daily Renewal Complex -Internal- Murad Pure Skin Clarifying Supplement	Murad Essential-C Daily Renewal Complex
EVENING	Murad Age Spot and Pigment Lightening Gel (Alternate)	Murad Essential-C Daily Renewal Complex (Alternate)	Murad Age-Balancing Night Cream -Internal- Murad Calming Nighttime Supplement	Murad Exfoliating Acne Treatment Gel -Internal- Murad Pure Skin Clarifying Supplement, as needed. Do not take with Murad Daily Renewal Complex Antioxidant Supplement or Murad Youth Builder Collagen Supplement	Murad Skin Smoothing Treatment

THIRTEEN

Internal Skin Care

Every morning and evening when you follow each step of your daily skin care program, some of the steps you are doing are basic maintenance, such as cleansing or moisturizing. What makes them different is that they incorporate my anti-aging recipe, ingredients that also hydrate, fight free radicals, and reduce inflammation while you're cleansing, toning, or hydrating. But the step that really delivers the active therapeutic punch of all three plus helps to build and repair collagen is the treat-and-repair step. The supplements you take are the internal treat-and-repair step.

You want to eat a healthy diet with a balance of protein, carbohydrates, and the right kinds of fats. But to really maximize your health, you want to include in that basic three as many fruits and vegetables and healthy fatty acids as you can. For reasons I'll soon explain, I think that the majority of us also need to take a multivitamin to maintain our health. In addition we need an extra dose of antioxidants, anti-inflammatory agents, collagen builders, and certain other nutrients to keep all of our cells healthy and our connective tissue—particularly our skin—strong and well hydrated.

In studies I've conducted measuring the effects of certain supplement formulas on skin, I've found that given the right raw materials, you can boost the power of your sunscreen, diminish cellulite, reduce wrinkles, improve acne, and improve stretch marks. But before learning which supplements can be used to treat and repair your skin, you need a well-balanced multivitamin as a kind of nutritional insurance. Of course I think you need to eat a healthy diet, but as conscientious as you try to be, it's very difficult to consistently get the basic nutrients you need to not only prevent deficiencies and disease but to help all your body functions perform at their maximum efficiency.

WELL-FED BUT UNDERNOURISHED

After years of assuring Americans that their diets are nutritionally adequate, nutritional experts are recognizing that many of us eat less than ideal diets for good health. It's unlikely we will develop scurvy, beriberi, or other deficiency conditions, but we may be at risk for what are called suboptimal levels of vitamins. And consuming too little of certain vitamins and minerals increases our risk of cancer, heart disease, osteoporosis, and prematurely aging skin.

Several surveys have shown that while we may be overfed, we're not necessarily well nourished. According to one report, the majority of women don't consume enough B vitamins, and half of us consume less than the recommended daily allowance of vitamins E and A, all of which are important vitamins for healthy skin. A third of us don't get enough vitamin C, which is essential for fighting free radicals and collagen production. Those at highest risk for suboptimal nutrition are women of childbearing age, vegetarians, people over sixty, people on weight-loss diets, and those taking certain drugs (see chart on page 177) or who drink more than two alcoholic beverages a day.

VITAMIN C: THE FRAGILE NUTRIENT

- The vitamin C content of apples falls by 67 percent after only two to three months of being picked.
- Potatoes harvested in the fall lose about two-thirds of their vitamin C by spring and all of it by summer.
- Green vegetables lose all their vitamin C within days of being stored at room temperature.
- Oranges lose 30 percent of vitamin C after squeezing.
- Freezing fruits and vegetables diminishes vitamin C by 25 percent.

And even if you do make an effort to eat healthy foods, you may not be getting all the nutrients the nutritional charts say those foods deliver. Even the 20 to 30 percent of Americans who make the effort to consistently eat the recommended five servings of fruits and vegetables a day may not be getting the vitamins and minerals they think their healthy eating guarantees. The amount of vitamins you get from foods depends on where they're grown, how fresh they are, how they've been stored, and how you cook them. For instance, if you keep food hot for more than two hours before you eat it, you're getting 10 percent less vitamin C, folate, and vitamin B_6. If you're one of those busy people who likes to cook ahead and you store your food in the refrigerator to reheat later, your fruits and vegetables will have 30 percent less vitamin C and folate than if you eat it fresh. Do you eat organic vegetables and fruits? There's evidence that they deliver more nutrients than those grown conventionally. For instance, organically grown oranges contain up to 30 percent more vitamin C than nonorganic ones that are twice the size.

Then, too, there are situations or conditions that affect how much you can absorb. For example, studies have shown that about one in five people over sixty have too little gastric acid to allow them to absorb vitamin B_{12} from food. If you're a woman over fifty, you need twice the vitamin D that you did when you were younger. Even if you drink D-fortified milk, you're only getting a quarter of the amount needed for calcium absorption in each cup. As for calcium, women over fifty and men over sixty-five need 1200 to 1500 mg of calcium a day. Now the prestigious National Academy of Sciences recommends that women who may become pregnant need to take a multivitamin with 400 micrograms of folic acid to avoid birth defects in their children. The Institute of Medicine, which establishes guidelines for healthy people, has said that smokers need 35 mg more of vitamin C a day than nonsmokers, because of the free radicals created by the habit.

Consuming enough of the essential fatty acids isn't easy, either. Do you typically eat three or four servings of cold-water fish each week? Are the fish farmed or wild? And if you do, are you certain that the fish are healthy and not high in toxins and mercury? Are you grinding up flaxseed to sprinkle on your cereal every day? Do you use walnut oil on your salad?

Considering all the factors that are known to affect our individual nutrient needs, we can only imagine about the unknown. Who knows how many more antioxidants are needed to combat the free radicals created by pollution, stress, and other causes of inflammation? And despite the fact that there are reams of published scientific papers on the antioxidant benefits of beta-carotene, there is still no official recommendation for how much is needed to counter the effects of living in a polluted environment.

DRUGS THAT MAY INTERFERE
WITH ABSORPTION

- Tetracycline interferes with absorption of calcium, magnesium, and iron.
- Many antibiotics interfere with absorption of B vitamins.
- Hormones, including oral contraceptives, reduce levels of some water-soluble vitamins.
- Antacids often coat the stomach and prevent calcium absorption.
- Vitamin C is poorly absorbed in the presence of aspirin, acetaminophen, and cortisone.
- Carbonated soft drinks interfere with calcium absorption.

We don't know precisely what extra nutrient demands are created by sun exposure, exercise, inflammation, pollution, and many other aspects of our lifestyle. How much vitamin A is needed to treat acne? What nutrients strengthen the skin's barrier so that eczema or excessive skin dryness don't occur? The best that we can do, I believe, is take supplemental nutrients in amounts that are greater than we can easily consume in the food we eat, but not so much that we create imbalances or reach toxic levels.

There is ample scientific evidence that providing extra nutrition in the form of supplements helps counteract the cell damage that results from free radical injury and inflammation. And, as you have learned in previous chapters, my own research has shown that supplying the body with extra nutrients reduces fine lines, increases the elasticity of the skin, helps build connective tissue, and increases the protective power of sunscreens.

I'm not suggesting that supplements replace foods, especially since fruits and vegetables are such a good source of fiber. I am recommending that you take supplements to lift yourself out of "suboptimal" nutrition to a healthier level of optimal nutrition. And then, if you want to treat your skin internally, I suggest that you take specific nutrients to counter the effects of aging on your skin and modify other conditions that are affecting your skin. While healthy people can tolerate these substances very well, and the dosages are safe, it's always a good idea to discuss any medication or extra nutrient supplements that you are taking with your physician. It's especially important if you are taking other prescription medications, if you are pregnant or planning on trying to conceive, or if you are having surgery.

START WITH A MULTIVITAMIN

Most multivitamins contain 100 percent or more of the daily value of vitamins A, B_1 (thiamin), B_2 (riboflavin), B_3 (niacin), B_6, B_{12}, C, D, and K. The Food and Nutrition Board of the National Academy of Sciences determined the amount sufficient to meet the nutrient requirements of most people.

Some multivitamins also contain minerals, such as calcium, but they may not be enough to meet your needs. For instance, typically a multivitamin contains 40 to 160 mg of calcium, but if you're a woman past menopause or a man over sixty-five, you may need ten times as much.

BOLSTER YOUR SUPPLY OF ANTIOXIDANTS

In 1996, I formulated the Murad Daily Renewal Complex Antioxidant Supplement, and seeing the improvements in my patients confirmed my belief that supplying the skin with extra antioxidants helped reverse the visible signs of aging. The formula I designed was not simply a booster dose of vitamin C—though that is one of the main ingredients in the formula. Rather, my antioxidant supplement combined nutrients and herbs that would be more powerful in protecting all layers of the skin from inflammation and free radical damage than any single component alone. This synergistic formula contains more than twenty-five wrinkle-fighting ingredients. In addition to a potent mix of antioxidant vitamins A, C, and E and carotenoids, among the ingredients the formula includes are:

- grape seed extract, a proanthocyanidin like pomegranate, which protects vital organs from free radical damage
- quercetin, an antioxidant and anti-inflammatory flavonoid that also works with vitamin C to build connective tissue
- silymarin, an antioxidant in milk thistle that targets the liver
- ginkgo biloba, an antioxidant especially active in the brain
- zinc, an essential trace mineral that is involved in the production of proteins and cell membranes. Zinc also works with the natural antioxidant enzyme superoxide dismutase
- lecithin, a chemical cousin of vitamin B, maintains the cell membrane
- cysteine, an amino acid that supports collagen building
- copper, an essential trace mineral that is involved in strengthening collagen
- yellow dock, an herb that reduces inflammation

- bupleurum, an herb that improves liver function
- gentian root, an herb that supports the liver
- myrrh, a natural gum that improves circulation
- hawthorn berry, a source of vitamin C
- wild yam, which contains hormones that the body converts to an anti-inflammatory hormone
- marshmallow root, which reduces inflammation

I recommend taking the Murad Daily Renewal Complex Antioxidant Supplement twice a day. If you are already taking an extra antioxidant supplement, you can check its contents against the formula that I recommend, which is provided in the appendix. You may want to add some other supplements to the one you're already taking to create your own supplement plan.

I suggest that anyone who is frequently exposed to the sun also take Murad Pomphenol Sunguard Supplement, a pomegranate supplement, to boost the effectiveness of sunscreen and fight free radicals. See "The Power of Pomegranate" on page 114.

I also recommend a twice-a-day supplement of 30 mg of coenzyme Q 10 if it is not in your multivitamin or other supplements (see chapter 6 for details on this potent antioxidant). If you are taking L-carnitine, you should take less coenzyme Q 10.

YOUTH BUILDER: A WRINKLE-FIGHTING PILL

When I formulated the Murad Youth Builder Collagen Supplement in 1996, my objective was to combine several anti-aging components that would create an ideal internal environment for building collagen. By maintaining the integrity of collagen and other connective tissues excessive water loss would also be prevented. I included antioxidants and anti-inflammatory nutrients to preserve the collagen and elastin that was already healthy, but I also included the basic building blocks that fibroblasts need to make new ones. I included certain minerals that promote connective tissue growth and protect the fibroblasts from injury. In addition to vitamins A, B_6, C, and E and beta-carotene, which is converted to vitamin A in the body, the formula contains:

- niacinamide, a derivative of niacin, or vitamin B_3, which is needed by cells to metabolize other nutrients, such as fatty acids and amino acids
- zinc, an essential trace mineral that is involved in the production of proteins and cell membranes. Zinc also works with the natural antioxidant enzyme superoxide dismutase to disarm free radicals and as an anti-inflammatory.
- selenium, an essential trace mineral and a powerful antioxidant
- copper, an essential trace mineral that is involved in strengthening collagen
- glucosamine, a building block of GAGs, which nourish the fibroblasts that make collagen and elastin
- grape seed extract, a proanthocyanidin like pomegranate, which protects vital organs from free radical damage
- amino acids, which are building blocks for the protein needed to build collagen and elastin
- quercetin, an antioxidant and anti-inflammatory flavonoid that also works with vitamin C to build connective tissue

Studies by an independent laboratory proved that my concept of rebuilding collagen worked. Women who took two tablets twice a day of my Youth Builder Collagen Supplement had a statistically significant 34 percent reduction in wrinkles and fine lines and an 18 percent increase in elasticity after five weeks.

Another study done by an independent laboratory confirmed my belief that the benefits of a collagen-building supplement aren't limited to the face. Thirty-seven women took Murad Youth Builder Plus, a modified form of the Youth Builder Collagen Supplement, for eight weeks, and another group took placebo pills. Those in the placebo group had a significant loss of elasticity in the skin of their thighs; those taking Murad Youth Builder Plus had no loss of elasticity. Despite the fact that those in the treatment group had not lost weight, they had a 78 percent increase in firmness of the skin of their thighs. They had a 13 percent improvement in the smoothness of cellulite and a 20 percent improvement in skin texture. After eight weeks, those taking Murad Youth Builder Plus also had a 25 percent improvement in the smoothness of their stretch marks and a 47 percent improvement in texture. Their stretch marks also got shorter, decreasing in length by 24 percent. Although there is still no cure for stretch marks, this study shows that they can be diminished with collagen-building supplements.

I believe that insuring that the body has all the nourishment it needs to build connective tissue doesn't just benefit the skin. In fact, many people with arthritis take the collagen builder glucosamine and have found it improves their joint symptoms. A study published in the British medical journal *The Lancet* found that people who took a daily dose of 1500 mg of glucosamine had 20 to 25 percent less pain than those taking a placebo. X rays of their joints showed that their arthritis had either stayed the same or improved, while those who took the placebo lost cartilage. At this point, we can only speculate that glucosamine, amino acids, and other collagen-building nutrients improve connective tissue throughout the body. But to me, it seems reasonable to assume that if the skin and cartilage benefit, then muscle, blood vessels, and other organs improve as well.

HELP SKIN HOLD WATER

Americans are becoming a nation of salmon eaters as word spreads of the heart-saving, cancer-preventing benefits of omega-3 fatty acids found in coldwater fish. With baby boomers graying fast, and their concerns shifting to preventing heart disease, omega-3's are the vitamin C of the new century. There are about forty books touting the benefits of omega-3's and how to get them in print today. Health newsletters, newspapers, and magazines provide a consistent flow of information on how to get more omega-3's into your daily diet.

The stir about omega-3 fatty acids is due to the fact that they reduce cholesterol and inflammation associated with heart disease, improve transmission of impulses in the brain, and defend against cancer. I agree that eating more cold-water fish (salmon, mackerel, herring, sardines), walnut oil, flaxseed, and a Mediterranean diet that relies on olive oil instead of butter is the ideal way to get not only omega-3's but other essential fatty acids as well. But knowing how difficult it is for people to get consistently adequate doses of any nutrient, I recommend an essential fatty acid supplement twice a day. In fact, the clinical studies that have proved the health benefits of omega-3 fatty acids used capsules, not fish, to deliver standardized doses.

A supplement of omega-3 fatty acids is insurance against the days that you don't eat fatty fish, and it allows you to consistently counter inflammation throughout your body. Also, I believe that since fatty acids are integral to the membranes surrounding your cells, keeping your body fully supplied with fatty acids maintains the integrity of your cell walls. And, as you now realize, strong cell walls mean cells don't lose water.

Most fish oil capsules and liquids contain two polyunsaturated omega-3 fatty acids: eicosapentaenoic acid (EPA) and docosahexaenoic acid (DHA). The typical supplement contains 18 percent EPA and 12 percent DHA. Both of these omega-3's have powerful anti-inflammatory effects and keep the pro-inflammatory omega-6 fatty acids in balance. To get the omega-3 fatty acid called linolenic acid, though, you have to eat leafy greens and walnut, flaxseed, or canola oil, though a few omega-3 supplements do contain linoleic acid as well.

The standard doses of omega-3's in fish oil capsules should not cause any side effects, but if you develop diarrhea, nausea, and a bad taste in your mouth, cut back on your daily dose.

Supplemental lecithin, phosphatidylcholine, and choline are also a kind of insurance, which is why I include them in Murad Wet Suit Hydrating Supplement. Although reports of deficiencies are uncommon, and the body itself manufactures them, I believe that a continually abundant supply of these cell-membrane building blocks insures that damage to the cell wall from inflammation and free radicals can be quickly repaired.

Side effects are rare, so even though the multivitamin or B-complex vitamin you are already taking may contain these nutrients, another supplement should not cause a problem and may improve your memory. But be sure to check with your doctor before taking any supplements.

SUPPLEMENTS FOR SPECIAL CONCERNS

Just as there are optional external treatments that address specific skin problems, there are internal treat-and-repair supplements that address your special concerns. For example, in Murad Pure Skin Clarifying Supplement, there is vitamin A to help normalize the production of excess skin cells within the follicles that clog the pore. Vitamins B_1, B_2, B_3, and B_6 assist tissue growth and repair, and zinc helps reduce the inflammation of acne. I've also included antioxidants, such as grape seed extract, because the inflammation of acne creates free radicals, too. In a study of thirteen people with acne, an independent laboratory found that all of the subjects had a 55 percent decrease in the number of acne lesions after taking Murad Pure Skin Clarifying Supplement for forty-two days. Since Pure Skin is so potent, it should not be taken with the antioxidant or Youth Builder formulas. Rather, take Pure Skin alone when you are troubled by breakouts. When the acne has subsided, you can stop Pure Skin and resume the other supplements in the program.

For women whose skin problems appear to be related to menopause, I recommend Murad Calming Nighttime Supplement. In addition to soothing frayed nerves and helping prevent insomnia, it contains glucosamine to boost collagen production.

For skin that is extremely stressed, overworked, and overprocessed, I've combined the most potent nutrients I know of in Murad Vital Spark Energy Supplement. To encourage repair and restoration, I've included a range of B vitamins, glucosamine, and amino acids. Antioxidants vitamin C, coenzyme Q 10, pomegranate, and two new ones that are generating a lot of excitement in the scientific community, oregano and curcumin, are in the supplement. These fight the excessive free radicals that stressed city skin is exposed to. Zinc helps relieve inflammation. Essential fatty acids help with cell membrane repair and hydration. This is a powerful supplement for skin that is depleted by inner stress and outer neglect. It's to be taken as needed, not continually.

SUPPLEMENTS ARE INSURANCE

You know as well as I do that the best diet for your body and your skin is one that consists of plenty of fresh green leafy vegetables and fruits; cold-water, fatty fish; high-fiber peas and beans; and healthy fats. I know that this same healthy diet is also best for your skin. For years I've been encouraging clients and patients who want to reverse the age-related changes in their skin to eat this way. Now studies are proving me right. People who eat more green leafy vegetables and beans throughout their lives are less wrinkled than those who eat a lot of processed, high-fat, and refined carbohydrate foods. But I'm also realistic, and I know how harried and stressful our lives are.

I believe to maintain the healthiest level of hydration throughout the entire body, the cell membranes and the connective tissues must be supplied with all the nutrients they need. Supplements of hydrating, anti-inflammatory, antioxidant, collagen-building nutrients are essential.

You will see the supplements I recommend in the daily regimens. In the appendix is a chart of the individual nutrients and the suggested amounts, if you would like to incorporate my recommendations into the daily supplements you are already taking.

FOURTEEN

Inclusive Skin Care

When someone asks me, "Are you having a good day?" I say, of course, why should I have a bad day when I can have a good day?

When you look in the mirror, your eye may focus in on the fine lines around your eyes, the furrow between your brows, the folds of loose flesh under your jawline, a mottled or dull complexion, brown spots, and red lines. If I were to look at your face, I'd probably see those signs of aging, too. But I would also see if you're angry and hostile or happy and friendly. I'd see if you are upset or calm, if you are bored with life or passionately involved, if you're loved and loving or isolated and sad.

As a dermatologist I can look at your skin, prescribe a program to make it healthier from the inside and the outside, as well as take years from your face. But I know that even if I make your skin perfect and youthful, there are other aspects of your life—and your health—that are going to affect how well your skin ages, too. Those aspects are a combination of your emotional, social, and spiritual life.

The combination of caring for your inner well-being along

with following the program I recommend for internal and external skin care is what I call inclusive skin care. And I believe you must address all of the factors that affect your skin if you want it to be beautiful and radiate vitality and joy.

I believe that to look your best, your heart has to be functioning at its optimum level. Your liver has to be working well. Every neuron in your brain has to be firing right along. And it helps to have a positive attitude toward life, have loving relationships with other people, and feel passionate about what you do. My whole belief system is an inclusive approach to health. You cannot just take one element of health, you have to look at every aspect of it.

Yes. You can get rid of wrinkles. You can fight free radicals and inflammation. You can keep your skin flush with water so that it's moist, soft, and pliable. But all of this rejuvenation is not going to be enough—and you're not going to be satisfied with the improvement—if you can't project a vision of health.

It might be easy to dismiss this as one man's personal philosophy, but as with other health concepts that I've introduced over the past thirty years, research in many disciplines is revealing hard data to support my experience as a dermatologist.

THE MIND-SKIN CONNECTION

Skin is a sensory organ as well as our body's protective envelope. It is richly supplied with nerves that signal touch and temperature, that turn on and off our sweat glands, that tell us to pull away from something unpleasant and to yield to what feels good. The skin detects nuances in our environment and communicates that information to the brain.

The skin can also reflect messages transmitted within our nervous system through what Harvard University researchers have dubbed the neuro-immuno-cutaneous-endocrine network, or NICE.

Discovery of this network confirms that the function of the nerves, the immune system, the actions and reactions taking place in our glands (the endocrine system), and the health of our skin are interrelated. If there is a malfunction in one aspect of this network, other areas will be affected, too. In broader terms, it's a mind-skin link that reflects health as well as disease.

The two-way communication throughout this network is a chemical one: hormones, proteins, growth factors, and neurotransmitters carry the signals. As a group, these chemicals are called *neuropeptides*. For instance, studies in laboratory rats and in humans have shown that there is direct signaling in the skin between immune cells, Langerhans' cells, and nerves. Identifying the chemicals, or neuropeptides, that carry these messages confirmed for scientists that there was a mind-body connection in the skin.

Of course, people with various skin problems have long known there was an association between their feelings, particularly stress, and conditions like acne, herpes, eczema, roseacea, and psoriasis. In one survey of more than five thousand people with psoriasis, a third of those who responded felt stress was the reason behind the periodic flares of their illness.

You have probably experienced the mind-skin connection in a healthy way. Have you ever become flush with excitement? Have you broken out in a cold sweat when you've been frightened? Has your hair ever stood on end when something "touched" you emotionally? Have you blushed with embarrassment? These skin reactions in the hair follicles, blood vessels, and sweat glands are triggered when something affects your mind and emotions.

A BROADER VIEW OF THE BODY

Eastern medicine has long acknowledged the impact of the emotions on the body, and the mind-body approach that is so integral to Chinese medicine and Ayurvedic medicine has gradually seeped into so-called holistic medicine practiced in the West. Traditional allopathically trained M.D.s may have been slow to accept many of the alternative practices, but the lack of endorsement hasn't had much of an impact on what people actually do to improve their health and well-being. Over a decade ago, a survey found that Americans visited alternative practitioners 40 million more times than they visited their primary care doctors. And since the 1990s, scores of American medical schools have developed "complementary medicine" departments that aim to incorporate some nontraditional practices, such as acupuncture and homeopathy, into the curriculum.

In research, too, scientists are finding that anxiety, stress, depression, and fear can affect health. Studies of gum disease, for example, have found that when people are under financial stress and lack the ability to cope with the strain, their risk of developing gum infection and inflammation doubles. Why should the skin, which is a very similar type of tissue, not respond to anxiety, stress, or depression?

Other research has shown that depression is linked to poor outcomes from heart surgery and spinal surgery. Fear, anxiety, and depression have also been associated with increased postoperative pain after gum surgery. And several studies have shown that stressful life events can contribute to acne and dry, itchy skin.

It's no longer unusual to see research published in prestigious, peer-reviewed medical journals confirming the molecular effects of some of the nontraditional practices. In a study of hypnosis following sun exposure, for example, Danish researchers found that people could decrease blood flow to their skin, which normally increases during inflammation. In another study, Cornell University researchers found that stress and sleep deprivation in women not only raised the level of stress hormones in the body, as they expected, it also had a negative impact on the skin's barrier function and increased water loss from the skin.

SKIN SUPPORT

It seems logical to me that if negative mental states and habits can cause disease, then positive attitudes, life-enhancing relationships, and therapies and treatments that make people feel good and help them relax could improve the body's function. If the mind can counter unhealthy inflammatory reactions, why can't it encourage healthy processes? I always recommend that my patients include some type of stress-reduction into their anti-aging, wrinkle-fighting program. I believe that like supplements, some types of relaxation therapy help boost the skin's health from the inside. You may need to do some experimenting to find a way of relaxing that works for you. For some women, having a manicure and hand and arm massage every week is relaxing. Some people—men, too—enjoy soaking in a fragrant bath surrounded by scented candles. They say it helps them destress at the end of a day. Quiet time for meditating in silence or listening to soothing music just a few minutes a day is centering for others. Whether it's giving yourself a facial or a foot massage, try to discover something that you can do routinely that encourages you to let go of tension.

In the Murad Spa, clients may have a facial not just to treat their skin but also to help them relax and benefit from being touched. A massage is another popular stress fighter. And some type of aromatherapy accompanies most treatments. Scientists looking at two potentially pleasurable sensations—touch and smell—are proving that I'm on the right track.

Aromatherapy. The scent of an essential oil is transferred by specialized nerves from the top of the nasal passages to the part of the brain that controls heart rate, memory, hormone balance, and other functions. Even scents so subtle that they are hard to identify have been found to stimulate a neurochemical response. Further indication that there is a connection between the nose and the brain is the finding that people who have a poor sense of smell are more likely to develop Alzheimer's disease, schizophrenia, and depression.

Essential oils massaged into the skin have been used for medicinal purposes in India, China, and the Middle East for centuries. But it wasn't until the 1930s that the science of aromatherapy was initiated in France. A chemist in the perfume industry accidentally burned himself and plunged his hand immediately into a vat of lavender oil. When he witnessed how quickly his injury healed, he began to study the regenerative value of essential oils.

It's believed that when essential oils are diffused in the bath or massaged on the skin, the body tissues absorb the molecules and that they have a therapeutic effect, especially on inflammatory conditions and infections, both of which involve the immune system.

Healing Touch. Another area of active research is touch therapy. Obviously, massage has a direct effect on the muscles and tissues that are being vigorously rubbed and stretched, but massage also relaxes the body, releases tension, and relieves pain. Studies conducted by the Touch Research Institute in Miami indicate that massage therapy can induce weight gain in premature infants and in adults and children with medical problems. It also alleviates depression, reduces stress hormones, alleviates pain, and positively alters the immune system.

There are various disciplines of what is called bodywork, which includes massage, deep-tissue manipulation, connective-tissue massage, reflexology, acupressure, and many more. So finding a "touch" therapy that works for you is easy. Even a fifteen-minute chair massage will help you relax and increase your alertness.

No doubt as research uncovers more biochemical connections between the skin, the brain, the immune system, and the glands, evidence that these systems can be stimulated and suppressed by forces like touch, fragrance, light, and sound will also be revealed.

DIFFERENT STROKES

I think that just as we know one antioxidant or anti-inflammatory agent alone cannot rejuvenate the skin, we'll learn that there is no single best method for diffusing stress or relieving tension, increasing energy, and improving mood. As I learned over the years of incorporating many of these treatments into my practice and at the Murad Spa, people can select from a menu of choices that works best for them. Some people's entire sense of well-being is improved by a good massage, others respond best when a specific weakness is addressed with acupuncture. Aromatherapy is a great tension reliever for some people, and yet others find the scents a bit overwhelming.

Only you know what works best for you. I encourage my patients and clients at the Murad Spa to try several alternative therapies and pay attention to what enhances their sense of well-being. Some women love the swaddled-like-a-baby comfort of an aromatherapy wrap; others feel claustrophobic and want to be unwrapped immediately. Most women love the relaxation of a professional facial almost as much as its skin-restoring benefits. Others become impatient and would much rather take a yoga class and stretch their way to relaxation and give themselves a facial at home.

The point is to have choices. To experiment and explore, and decide what you like. I can recommend treatments based on my knowledge and professional experience, but only you know if what I or anyone else suggests is helpful for you. That's one reason why I provide optional treatments in my anti-aging program that you can alternate or use instead of the recommended treat-and-repair step. If you limit your choices you don't have the ability to have the best outcome.

THE WELLNESS EXPERIENCE

There have been attempts recently to bring the spa into the dermatologist's or plastic surgeon's office and the doctor into the spa. I realized in the mid-1980s, when I first included an esthetician in my dermatology practice and opened my first spa, A Sense of Self, and later when I asked an acupuncturist and a nutritionist to join me, that to satisfy the needs of my patients, more than one discipline was required. Eventually, I designed the Murad Spa in Los Angeles in order to fully develop my concept of inclusive skin care. I believe that the spa environment is the future wellness facility. In many ways it's already happening, as people's desire for an inclusive approach to wellness has contributed to the booming spa industry. Spas are now providing many of the treatments that address the underlying lifestyle-related causes of disease, such as stress, poor nutrition, lack of exercise, and isolation.

Today health and beauty really can come together in the spa. It's an inclusive approach to health that acknowledges how important appearance is to a person's sense of well-being. Feeling good about one's appearance is, I think, as important as being fit and well nourished. In fact, a person who is active, eating a well-balanced diet, taking supplements, and in control over life's stresses also looks good. And all of these healthy habits help counter inflammation, which is the cause of many chronic diseases and signs of aging.

A PASSION FOR LIFE

Of course, if coping with the stresses of life were as simple as putting some aromatic essential oils in the bath, we wouldn't have chronic stress-related diseases and so many people wouldn't appear much older than their years. I think it's just as important to care for your emotional and spiritual life as it is to exercise, take the right vitamins, and follow my skin care program. To me, caring for yourself also means examining your life and doing what you can to make it better. Ultimately, the best stress reliever is not to have any stress. And having healthy relationships with others, being involved in things that matter to you, and enjoying time to relax and refresh help you create a life that encourages health.

One of the major "diseases" of our society today, I think, is isolation. Too many of us work too hard, spend too much time alone, and have too few connections to others. Of course, you can't tell a person who seems lonely and uncared for and somewhat depressed to go out and make friends. But what I try to do is encourage people to find something about which they can feel passionate. It may be an intellectual pursuit or work-related interest, but it could just as well be smelling roses or watching birds or hiking. Then, through pursuing their passion, they can join organizations that will put them in touch with others who share their passion. The connection to others, then, is natural and caring and will evolve in those who are open to it. If fear of rejection is stopping you, be brave and try to be open to opportunities.

To help counter the day-to-day stresses over which you have no control—like a traffic jam on the freeway—you need a let-it-be attitude. It may be appropriate to get angry at the driver who cut

FINDING A CONNECTION

Being part of a community isn't just about taking encouragement and help from others; it's also about giving and being responsive to others. A patient of mine, Daphne, created a community almost in spite of herself.

As her children were growing up, Daphne was a full-time mother. And like most suburban women married to husbands who frequently traveled, most of the parenting chores were hers. She enjoyed her life, even though having three children very close in age kept her too busy to join friends for afternoon tennis or bridge games.

When Daphne's last child left home for college, though, she found herself with more free time than she was accustomed to. Unfortunately, she also began to be troubled by various health problems. Her back hurt, and she had frequent headaches and chronic shoulder pain. Playing tennis was out, but she did meet her old friends for lunch occasionally even though she didn't feel she had much in common with them. One day, she passed by a yoga studio and was reminded that she had always wanted to try it.

After the first class, Daphne felt she had found something that had been missing from her life. She loved the physical exertion, the sensation of feeling her own strength, and the peaceful relaxed feeling that followed. She started going several times a week and reading about the different styles of yoga. Yoga quickly became a passion for her.

The downside was that she felt a little out of place, since she was so much older than the twenty-something women who regularly attended the classes. But her interest in yoga was stronger than her awkwardness about her age, so she kept going. Gradually, Daphne began talking with the others before and after class, and then was invited to join a group of them for tea afterward. That was the beginning of what became deep friendships . . . and a sense of community.

Daphne has become a kind of mother to the group. They respect her experience, and she often finds herself helping those who live far from their own families. Sometimes it's just being a willing listener. Sometimes it's advice on coping with a child's behavior problems, or teaching some of the women how to cook. Since Daphne's become part of this community, she has become more youthful looking. Part of it, I'm sure, is the result of her regular yoga practice, but I also think her brightness and energy are because she's no longer so isolated.

---

you off or the friend who betrayed your trust, but harboring the anger and resentment won't help you and doesn't improve the situation. The inner turmoil takes a toll on your health and your looks. If you can't do something about the situation, then let it go.

On the other hand, when you do have the power to change a situation, do it. If you are miserable in your job, start trying to find a new one. Massage and aromatherapy will help ease your way, but you've got to make the change yourself. You may make less money, you may have to move, but how does the stress of

PYRAMID OF HEALTH

Beautiful skin is a reflection of health that encompasses a person's physical, emotional, and spiritual well-being. The foundation—the base of the pyramid—is the absence of disease. When illness or injury does occur, prompt, state-of-the-art treatment is imperative, for without a solid healthy foundation, everything else is weakened.

A sense of well-being, the next level of the pyramid, is a balance between the many aspects of your emotional life and a healthy, self-caring lifestyle. It includes having passion and caring in your life, reducing isolation with strong connections to other people, intimate relationships, a loving attitude that's free of hostility and anger, and a feeling of satisfaction that you're using your talents well. Self-caring means that you treat your body with respect: you exercise, get enough sleep, and take time to relax.

The next step of the pyramid is fueling your healthy mind and body with supplements for energy, growth, and renewal. Supplements are also needed to maintain your defenses against harmful environmental factors and internal inflammation.

Finally, and at the top of the pyramid, is healthy eating. And by this I don't mean following a list of must-haves and don'ts. My idea of healthy eating is to eat a variety of foods and listen to your body's signals. It will let you know in many ways when you're not getting the right nutrients, enough water, or enough calories. Learn to know the dif-

ference between craving and real hunger. Most important
is to avoid deprivation, which I think will only drive you to
eat more of what you think you are missing.

---

accommodating yourself to something you care about compare to
the stress of being trapped in a miserable situation?

It's become widely accepted now that many people who are
facing emotional or physical crises benefit from being part of a
healing community. It can be a formal support group or a loose
circle of friends and family. Even the personal exchanges at the
hair salon or barbershop give some people a chance to share their
feelings and concerns with another supportive person. But I
believe that even when a crisis isn't looming, being part of a community enhances well being. Certainly we know that the reverse—
isolation—contributes to poor health.

When I see men and women whose deeply lined faces make
them appear haggard, defeated, sorrowful, and older than their
years, I try to encourage them to try to find the thing that will
make them feel passionate and do it. Many people who appear
angry or sad are not able to recognize their own potential. It's the
reverse of the cartoon that shows the pussycat looking in the mirror and seeing the lion. Too often, it's the lion looking in the mirror
and seeing a pussycat. We all have it within us to do more. What
holds us back is our lack of belief in our own strength and power.

SELF-CARE

Today, when people come to me because of a skin condition like
acne or eczema, instead of just writing a prescription for an
antibiotic or an anti-inflammatory cream, I ask them to tell me

about how they care for themselves. Do they exercise? What do they eat? What is their work like? And with all due respect to their privacy, I ask if they are having any particular strain or stress in their lives or in their relationships?

As a physician, I believe that getting a true picture of my patients' quality of life is as important in planning their treatment as accurately diagnosing the condition affecting their skin. Of course, my first concern is to treat their skin problem, but then I'll also help them design a supplement plan for nutritional support and a mind-body treatment—aromatherapy, acupuncture, massage, or some other supportive therapy—that will enhance their immune response. By treating the whole person in this way, I think I improve not only their skin condition but their overall health as well.

One thing I always try to avoid is adding more stress to their lives. This often happens when people go to the doctor and are told, for instance, that they must lose weight. Or that they have to eat this fish every day and no carbohydrates. Or only leafy greens and no potatoes or desserts. Obviously, nutrition plays a crucial role in health, and most Americans are eating far too many calories, but I have never seen any diet that really works long-term. Weight-loss diets especially, in my opinion, are a setup for failure. Not only do most people regain the weight they lose, they've often put themselves through weeks of stress and deprivation that only creates more internal havoc. In an attempt to get healthy, they've become more anxious and unhappy, and coping with these unpleasant emotions takes a toll on their skin.

One young patient of mine didn't begin to lose weight until she gave up on diets. After seeing her weight go up and down like a yo-yo, she decided to be conscious of eating healthy foods, but not to deprive herself if she felt she really had to have a particular food. Her weight loss has been slower than the temporary losses she had with diets in the past, but she's still losing—and not regaining.

Instead of dieting, I talk to my patients about trying to listen harder to their body and to pay attention to what they eat and why. The most important thing for most of us to learn is what true hunger feels like, and to let that sensation—not a clock or a special diet—dictate what we eat. Eating slowly is also helpful because it helps people tune into the pleasure of their sense of smell and taste. Also, it gives the brain time to know when the stomach is full. Eating slowly and with complete awareness of what is going into your mouth allows you to eat what you need to feel satisfied and no more. It takes practice and patience, but long-term you'll naturally eat less and more healthily. Taking supplements is part of this plan, too.

In addition to learning what you find relaxing and restorative, you also need to pay attention to what's going on in your body and your physical and emotional environment. Just as you modify your skin care program as your skin changes, so your body's needs may change with the seasons, your hormonal shifts, and the pressures and pleasures of your life. I don't think checking in with yourself on a weekly basis is too often to pay attention to how you're really feeling. Think of it like stepping on the scale to check your weight. How is your general mood? Your energy level? Your sense of your physical self? Just as you peer at yourself in the mirror to search for new lines and wrinkles, check your emotional temperature. Are you feeling satisfied, challenged, cared about by those you care for? Have you spent any time sharing and giving to others?

SKIN CARE IS HEALTH CARE

When I lecture around the country, I often talk about how skin care is health care. If I can heal your skin and help it to become as healthy and vital as possible, I'm also helping you improve the health of your whole body. Doing everything you can to improve the water-holding capacity of your skin improves all the cells of your body. Protecting your skin and its immune cells from the damaging rays of the sun helps to defend your entire immune system. Taking supplements to improve the quality of the connective tissue of your skin also improves the connective tissue wherever it exists in your body.

During the 1990s we saw an increase in so-called new-age drugs that improved the quality of one's life. We have Propecia to help grow hair, Viagra to help men overcome sexual difficulties, and a plethora of mood-altering drugs to help overcome everything from shyness to depression. And we can now take a supplement to reduce wrinkles, protect against sun damage, and to revitalize our skin. We're beginning to learn how to alter our body chemistry with alternative treatments and live to our fullest potential. It's as if the newest pharmacological approaches to looking good and enjoying life have joined with age-old healing therapies.

The next step in what I call inclusive skin care will be an environment where health care practitioners will be partners. The team will include estheticians, acupuncturists, body workers, and nutritionists. This will be a caring and compassionate atmosphere that will allow people to achieve optimum health—a sense of satisfaction with their present life and the ability to accomplish what they want.

We are each born with a unique commodity

called life. It is stressed by the environment,

and it is up to us to make the best of it.

—*Howard Murad, MD*

Appendix

Note: This appendix begins with detailed tables listing the ingredients in Murad products (pages 205–214). The supplements are patented formulas that are essential to your internal skin care program. The appendix continues with our "What to Look for Guide," a series of charts listing products available from drugstores, salons, spas, and department stores. The charts cover both Murad products and products from other manufacturers at a variety of price points (pages 215–232).

To obtain the products listed in the appendix, go to

www.murad.com or 1-800-33MURAD
www.sephora.com or 1-877-SEPHORA
www.nordstrom.com or 1-888-7BEAUTY
www.beauty.com
www.gloss.com
www.drugstore.com

Ingredients in Murad Internal Skincare

Murad Youth Builder Collagen Supplement

Supplement Facts		
Two tablets twice a day contain:	Amount Per Serving	% Daily Value
Vitamin A (Palmitate)	4000IU	80%
Vitamin B-3 (Niacinamide)	80mg	400%
Vitamin B-6 (Pyridoxine HCl)	20mg	1000%
Vitamin C (Magnesium Ascorbate)	400mg	667%
Vitamin E (D-alpha Tocopherol Succinate)	100IU	333%
N-Acetyl D-Glucosamine	160mg	*
L-Proline	360mg	*
L-Lysine (HCl)	320mg	*
Glucosamine Sulfate	1200mg	*
N-Acetyl Cysteine	120mg	*
Quercetin	80mg	*
Grape Seed Extract	30mg	*
Zinc (Opti-Zinc™ 24mg)	6mg	*
Magnesium (Ascorbate)	12mg	*
Copper (Sebacate)	1.6mg	*
Selenomethionine (L-Selenomethionine)	80mcg	*
Beet Root Powder	135mg	*
Essential Fatty Acid Complex (Oleic Acid, Linoleic Acid, Gamma Linoleic Acid, Alpha Linoleic Acid, Eicosapentaenoic Acid (EPA), Docahexaenoic Acid (DHA))	150mg	*
Phosphatidylcholine	45mg	*
L-Glycine	45mg	*
Inositol	45mg	*
Curcumin (from Tumeric)	45mg	*
*Daily Value not established.		

Other Ingredients: Dicalcium Phosphate, Microcrystalline Cellulose, Stearic Acid, Magnesium Stearate, Silica, Croscarmellose Sodium, Pharmaceutical Glaze, Talc.

Murad Daily Renewal Complex Antioxidant Supplement

Supplement Facts

Two tablets twice a day contain:	Amount Per Serving	% Daily Value
Vitamin A (as Palmitate)	2500IU	50%
Beta Carotene	1500IU	30%
Vitamin C (from Ascorbic Acid)	800mg	1033%
Vitamin E Natural	280IU	933%
Zinc Oxide	24mg	160%
Copper (chelate)	0.6mg	30%
Green Tea Extract	192mg	*
Echinacea Root Powder	192mg	*
Gentian Root Powder	192mg	*
Golden Seal Root Powder	192mg	*
Myrrh Gum	192mg	*
Poria Cocos (Fu Ling)	192mg	*
Milk Thistle Seed Extract (83% Silymarin)	158mg	*
N-Acetyl Cysteine	90mg	*
Rosemary Leaf Extract	160mg	*
Yellow Dock Root Powder	150mg	*
Glucosamine HCl	65mg	*
L-Glycine	75mg	*
Origanox™	100mg	*
Quercetin	85mg	*
Hawthorn Berry Extract	65mg	*
Choline	75mg	*
Wild Yam Root Powder	80mg	*
Bee Pollen	75mg	*
FoTi Root Powder	58mg	*
Royal Jelly Concentrate	25mg	*
Grape Seed Extract	20mg	*
Ginkgo Biloba Leaf Extract	4mg	*
Pomegranate Extract	5mg	*
Biotin	300mcg	*

Selenium (L-Selenomethionine)	80mcg	*
Lecithin	25mg	*
Curcumin (from Tumeric)	45mg	*
Essential Fatty Acid Complex (Oleic Acid, Linoleic Acid, Gamma Linoleic Acid, Alpha Linoleic Acid, Eicosapentaenoic Acid (EPA), Docahexaenoic Acid (DHA))	125mg	*
Phosphatidylcholine	45mg	*
Inositol	45mg	*
*Daily Value not established.		

Other Ingredients: Dicalcium Phosphate, Microcrystalline Cellulose, Stearic Acid, Magnesium Stearate, Silica, Croscarmellose Sodium, Pharmaceutical Glaze, Talc.

Murad Wet Suit Hydrating Supplement

Supplement Facts

Two tablets once a day contain:	Amount Per Serving	% Daily Value
Vitamin C	120mg	200%
Vitamin E (Acetate)	100mg	333%
Zinc	10mg	67%
Manganese	4mg	200%
Copper	2mg	100%
Selenium	150mcg	214%
Type II Collagen	250mg	*
Glucosamine Sulfate	170mg	*
Essential Fatty Acid Complex (Oleic Acid, Linoleic Acid, Gamma Linoleic Acid, Eicosapentaenoic Acid (EPA), Docahexaenoic Acid (DHA))	150mg	*
Dipotassium Phosphate	150mg	*
Choline	100mg	*
L-Lysine	90mg	*
L-Glycine	90mg	*
Aloe Vera Concentrate	60mg	*
Potassium Sulfate	50mg	*
Curcumin (from Turmeric)	35mg	*
Coenzyme Q 10	10mg	*
Pomegranate Extract (5% Ellagic Acid)	5mg	*
Phosphatidylcholine (from Lecithin)	1500mcg	*

Other Ingredients: Cellulose, Vegetable Stearate, Magnesium Stearate, Stearic Acid, Silica, Pharmaceutical Glaze, Talc.

Murad Pomphenol Sunguard Supplement

Supplement Facts		
One tablet per day contains:	**Amount Per Serving**	**% Daily Value**
Pomegranate (Punica granatum) Extract (5% Ellagic Acid)	15mg	*

Other Ingredients: Beet Juice Powder, Cellulose, Pharmaceutical Glaze.

Murad Pure Skin Clarifying Supplement

Supplement Facts

Two tablets twice a day contain:	Amount Per Serving	% Daily Value
Vitamin A (as Palmitate)	4000IU	80%
Beta Carotene	2500IU	25%
Vitamin B-1 (Thiamine HCl)	25mg	1666%
Vitamin B-2 (Riboflavin)	25mg	1470%
Vitamin B-3 (Niacin)	50mg	250%
Vitamin B-5 (Pantothenic Acid)	25mg	250%
Vitamin B-6 (Pyridoxine HCl)	50mg	2500%
Biotin	300mcg	100%
Vitamin C (Calcium 60% & Zinc Ascorbate 40%)	300mg	500%
Folic Acid	400mcg	100%
Vitamin E Natural	400IU	1333%
Calcium (Ascorbate)	62mg	6%
Magnesium (Oxide)	200mg	50%
Zinc (Ascorbate)	15mg	100%
Glucosamine HCl	65mg	*
L-Lysine HCl	250mg	*
L-Glycine	250mg	*
L-Proline	500mg	*
Alpha Lipoic Acid	50mg	*
Silica (Derived from 400mg Horsetail Leaf Extract)	28mg	*
Grape Seed Extract (38.4%)	50mg	*
Selenium (L-Selenomethionine)	200mcg	*
Lecithin	75mg	*
Essential Fatty Acid Complex (Oleic Acid, Linoleic Acid, Gamma Linoleic Acid, Alpha Linoleic Acid, Eicosapentaenoic Acid (EPA), Docahexaenoic Acid (DHA))	150mg	*
Burdock Root Powder	83mg	*
Yellowdock Powder	97mg	*

Chromium (as Picolinate)	100mcg	*
Pomegranate Extract	2mg	*
Origanox™	100mg	*
Aloe Vera Powder	75mg	*
Curcumin (from Tumeric)	45mg	*
Coenzyme Q 10	800mcg	*
*Daily Value not established.		

Other Ingredients: Dicalcium Phosphate, Microcrystalline
Cellulose, Stearic Acid, Magnesium Stearate, Croscarmellose
Sodium, Aerosil, Pharmaceutical Glaze, Talc.

Murad Vital Spark Energy Supplement

Supplement Facts

Two tablets as needed contain:	Amount Per Serving	% Daily Value
Vitamin B-1 (Thiamine HCl)	50mg	3333%
Vitamin B-2 (Riboflavin)	20mg	1176%
Vitamin B-3 (80 mg Niacinamide & 40 mg Niacin)	120mg	600%
Vitamin B-5 (D-Calcium Pantothenate)	120mg	1200%
Vitamin B-6 (Pyridoxine HCl)	25mg	1250%
Vitamin B-12 (Cyanocobalamin)	50mcg	833%
Folic Acid	400mcg	100%
Biotin	50mcg	17%
Vitamin C (Ascorbic Acid, Zinc, & Manganese Ascorbate)	150mg	250%
Magnesium (Oxide, Citrate)	120mg	30%
Potassium (Citrate)	99mg	*
Calcium (Citrate)	60mg	6%
Zinc (Ascorbate)	10mg	67%
Manganese (Ascorbate)	5mg	*
Essential Fatty Acid Complex (Oleic Acid, Linoleic Acid, Gamma Linoleic Acid, Alpha Linoleic Acid, Eicosapentaenoic Acid (EPA), Docahexaenoic Acid (DHA))	250mg	*
L-Glutamine	250mg	*
L-Tyrosine	225mg	*
DAME (Bitartrate)	150mg	*
L-Carnitine	100mg	*
L-Phenylalanine	100mg	*
Choline (Bitartrate)	100mg	*
Curcumin Powder	100mg	*
Glucosamine Sulfate HCl	65mg	*
Origanox™	100mg	*
L-Glycine	75mg	*
Ginkgo Biloba Leaf Extract	50mg	*

Lecithin	35mg	*
Inositol	30mg	*
Coenzyme Q 10	10mg	*
Pomegranate Extract (Ellagic Acid)	5mg	*
Phosphatidylcholine	350mcg	*
Herbal Formula	350mg	*
(Siberian Ginseng, 200 mg; Gotu Kola, 100 mg; Schizandra, 25 mg; Ginger Root, 25 mg; Raspberry Powder, 25 mg)		
*Daily value not established.		

Other Ingredients: Dicalcium Phosphate, Microcrystalline Cellulose, Magnesium Stearate, Silica, Hydroxypropyl Methylcellulose, Polyethylene Glycol, FD & C Red #40, FD & C Blue #1, Titanium Dioxide.

Warnings: Contains Phenylalanine. Not to be used by phenylketonurics, pregnant or nursing women, or with antidepressant drugs. If you have severe chronic high blood pressure, take immediately after meals and/or consult with your physician.

Murad Calming Nighttime Supplement

Supplement Facts

Two tablets in the evening contain:	Amount Per Serving	% Daily Value
Vitamin A (Acetate)	3000IU	60%
Vitamin B2 (Riboflavin)	20mg	1176%
Vitamin B6 (Pyridoxine)	30mg	1500%
Vitamin C	120mg	200%
Niacin (Niacinamide)	30mg	150%
Zinc (from Oxide, Sulfate, and Optizinc)	40mg	267%
Biotin	600mcg	600%
L-Arginine HCl	300mg	*
L-Alanine	200mg	*
L-Glycine	150mg	*
White Willow Bark (Powder)	200mg	*
Shark Cartilage (Powder)	200mg	*
Alpha Lipoic Acid	120mg	*
Pomegranate Extract (15% Ellagic Acid)	10mg	*
Curcumin (from Tumeric)	40mg	*
Melatonin	1mg	*
Glucosamine Sulfate	200mg	*
Origanox™	150mg	*
L-Carnitine	80mg	*
Essential Fatty Acids Complex	170mg	*
Coenzyme Q 10	1mg	*

Other Ingredients: Microcrystalline Cellulose, Dicalcium Phosphate, Croscarmellose Sodium, Stearic Acid, Magnesium Stearate.

THE WHAT TO LOOK FOR GUIDE

Product Name	Product Category	Hydrating, Antioxidant and Skin Soothing Ingredients *listed in the order as they appear on the product label
Murad Refreshing Cleanser	Cleanser Normal/Combination	Algae Extract, Hedychium Coronarium (White Ginger) Root Extract, Actinidia Chinensis (Kiwi) Fruit Extract, Cucumis Sativus (Cucumber) Fruit Extract, Citrus Aurantium Dulcis (Orange) Fruit Extract, Sodium PCA
Beauty Without Cruelty 3% Alpha Hydroxy Cleanser	Cleanser Normal/Combination	Orange Blossom Extract, Lavender, Aloe Vera Gel, Vegetable Glycerin, Lactic Acid, Allantoin, Tocopherol (Vitamin E), Retinyl Palmitate (Vitamin A), Ascorbic Acid (Vitamin C)
Garden Botanika Balancing Gel Cleanser	Cleanser Normal/Combination	Vitamin E, Aloe Vera Gel, Licorice Extract, Grape Seed Extract, Ginseng Extract, Green Tea Extract
Peter Thomas Roth Silky Cleansing Cream	Cleanser Normal/Combination	Sodium PCA, Chamomile Extract, Panthenol, Magnesium Ascorbyl Phosphate, Vitamins A & E

All of the products mentioned in this chart contain a hydrator, an antioxidant, and a skin soother. In some cases, they also contain additional active ingredients. The Murad product appears first, and other products follow. Since formulas and sources of ingredients vary widely, the effectiveness, safety, and cosmetic considerations may vary from one product to another. Also, in some people, using different brands of products may cause interactions that are unpredictable.

Product Name	Product Category	Hydrating, Antioxidant and Skin Soothing Ingredients
Murad Moisture Rich Cleanser	Cleanser Dry/Sensitive	Sodium PCA, Sorbitol, Algae Extract, Panthenol, Anthemis Nobilis Flower (Chamomile) Extract, Cucumis Sativus (Cucumber) Fruit Extract, Citrus Grandis (Grapefruit) Fruit Extract
Alba Botanica Citrus Cream Cleanser, Delicate Skin	Cleanser Dry/Sensitive	Chamomile, Almond Oil, Vegetable Glycerin, Jojoba Oil, Lime Tree and Burdock Root Extract, d-Alpha Tocopheryl (Vitamin E), Retinyl Palmitate (Vitamin A)
Osmotics Hydrating Cleanser	Cleanser Dry/Sensitive	Extracts of Kelp, Calendula, Ginkgo, Aloe Vera, Sambucus, Althea Horsetail, Glycerin, Sodium PCA, Tocopherol Acetate (Vitamin E), Retinyl Palmitate (Vitamin A), Ascorbic Acid (Vitamin C)
Murad Clarifying Cleanser	Cleanser Oily/Acne	Salicylic Acid, Cimicifuga Racemosa Root (Black Cohosh) Extract, Camellia Oleifera Leaf (Green Tea) Extract, Citrus Aurantium Amara (Bitter Orange) Oil, Lavandula Hybrida (Lavender) Oil, Prunus Armeniaca (Apricot Kernel) Oil
Cuticura Acne Treatment Foaming Face Wash with Salicylic Acid	Cleanser Oily/Acne	Salicylic Acid, Glycerin, Allantoin, Tocopheryl Acetate (Vitamin E), Aloe Vera

Product	Type / Skin	Ingredients
SkinScience Exfoclean Gentle AHA Cleanser	Cleanser Oily/Acne	Lavandula Angustifolia (Lavender) Oil, Panthenol, Salicylic Acid, Retinyl Palmitate (Vitamin A) Cholecalciferol (Vitamin B3), Vitamin E Acetate (Tocopheryl Acetate)
Murad AHA/BHA Exfoliating Cleanser	Exfoliating Cleanser	Simmondsia Chinensis (Jojoba) Seed Oil, Sodium PCA, Glycolic Acid, Lactic Acid, Salicylic Acid, Dipotassium Glycyrrhizate (Licorice Extract), Sodium Ascorbyl Phosphate (Vitamin C)
Ecco Bella Daily Exfoliant	Exfoliating Cleanser	Aloe Vera, Lemon and Passionfruit Acids, Lactic Acid, Salicylic Acid, Extracts of Oat, Calendula and Licorice, Essential Oils of Lavender, Rosemary and Geranium, Grapefruit Seed Extract
Murad Hydrating Toner	Toner Normal/Combination and Dry/Sensitive	Algae Extract, Prunus Persica (Peach) Fruit Extract, Sodium PCA, Tocopherol (Vitamin E), Magnesium Ascorbyl Phosphate (Vitamin C)
Skin Ceuticals Revitalizing Toner, Normal or Dry Skin	Toner Normal/Combination and Dry/Sensitive	Aloe Vera Gel, Mixed Fruit Extract, Glycerin, Allantoin, Panthenol, Chamomile Extract, Calendula Extract, Cucumber Extract

All of the products mentioned in this chart contain a hydrator, an antioxidant, and a skin soother. In some cases, they also contain additional active ingredients. The Murad product appears first, and other products follow. Since formulas and sources of ingredients vary widely, the effectiveness, safety, and cosmetic considerations may vary from one product to another. Also, in some people, using different brands of products may cause interactions that are unpredictable.

Product Name	Product Category	Hydrating, Antioxidant and Skin Soothing Ingredients
ORANGEDAILY Daily Toner, Non-Alcoholic Antioxidant Formula	Toner Normal/Combination and Dry/Sensitive	Methylsilanol Ascorbate (Vitamin C), Sodium PCA, Algae Extract, Glycerin, Camellia Oleifera (Green Tea) Extract, Phospolipids, Tangerine Oil
Murad Clarifying Toner	Toner Oily/Acne	Algae Extract, Cucumis Sativus (Cucumber) Fruit Extract, Citrus Medica Limonum (Lemon) Extract, Calendula Officinalis (Calendula) Flower Extract, Tocopherol (Vitamin E), Magnesium Ascorbyl Phosphate (Vitamin C), Allantoin, Vitis Vinifera (Grape) Seed Extract
Astara AHA Nutrient Toning Essence	Toner Oily/Acne	Aloe Vera, Calendula, Lactic Acid, Cucumber Extract, Sodium Hyaluronate, Ascorbic Acid (Vitamin C), Tocopheryl Acetate (Vitamin E), Panthenol
Beauty Without Cruelty Aroma-therapy Balancing Facial Toner	Toner Oily/Acne	Orange Blossom, Horsetail, Calendula, Elderflower, Chamomile, Sodium PCA, Aloe Vera Gel, Kelp, Algae Extract, Cucumber Extract, Vitamin E, Retinyl Palmitate (Vitamin A), Ascorbic Acid (Vitamin C)
Murad Essential-C Daily Renewal Complex	Antioxidant Treatment	Ascorbic Acid (Vitamin C), Tocopheryl Acetate (Vitamin E), Retinol (Vitamin A), Bisabolol (Chamomile), Allantoin, Zinc Aspartate, Retinyl Palmitate (Vitamin A), Beta-Carotene

Product	Type	Ingredients
Cellex-C Advanced-C Serum	Antioxidant Treatment	Ascorbic Acid, Zinc, Sodium Hyaluronate, Grape Skin Extract, Bioflavonoids
Peter Thomas Roth Power C Anti-Oxidant Serum Gel	Antioxidant Treatment	L-Ascorbic Acid (Vitamin C), Sodium Hyaluronate, Glycerin, Ginkgo Biloba, Green Tea Extract, Beta Glucan
Murad Combination Skin Treatment	Treatment Normal/Combination	Glycolic Acid, Aloe Barbadensis Leaf Juice, Salicylic Acid, Citrus Aurantium Dulcis (Orange) Fruit Extract, Zinc Aspartate, Sodium Hyaluronate, Tocopherol (Vitamin E), Magnesium Ascorbyl Phosphate (Vitamin C), Dipotassium Glycyrrhizate (Licorice Extract), Vitis Vinifera (Grape) Seed Extract, Zinc Acetate, Retinyl Palmitate (Vitamin A)
Estée Lauder Fruition Extra	Treatment Normal/Combination	Green Tea Extract, Salicylic Acid, Licorice Extract, Tocopheryl Acetate (Vitamin E), Sodium Hyaluronate, Retinyl Palmitate (Vitamin A), Phospholipids, Lavender
Z. Bigatti Re-Storation Skin Treatment Facial Lotion	Treatment Normal/Combination	Glycerin, Glycolic Acid, Salicylic Acid, Avocado Oil, Grape Seed Extract, Tocopheryl Acetate (Vitamin E), Hyaluronic Acid, Retinyl Palmitate (Vitamin A), Green Tea Extract, Panthenol

All of the products mentioned in this chart contain a hydrator, an antioxidant, and a skin soother. In some cases, they also contain additional active ingredients. The Murad product appears first, and other products follow. Since formulas and sources of ingredients vary widely, the effectiveness, safety, and cosmetic considerations may vary from one product to another. Also, in some people, using different brands of products may cause interactions that are unpredictable.

Product Name	Product Category	Hydrating, Antioxidant and Skin Soothing Ingredients
Murad Skin Smoothing Treatment SPF 8	Treatment Dry	Glycolic Acid, Zinc Aspartate, Sodium Hyaluronate, Aloe Barbadensis Leaf Juice, Tocopheryl Linolate (Vitamin E), Dipotassium Glycyrrhizate (Licorice Extract), Tocopherol, Magnesium Ascorbyl Phosphate (Vitamin C), Vitis Vinifera (Grape Seed Extract), Panthenol, Retinyl Palmitate (Vitamin A), Chamomilla Recutita (Matricaria) Flower Extract
Beauty Without Cruelty Aromatherapy 8% Alpha Hydroxy Complex Renewal Moisture Cream	Treatment Dry	Lavender, Meadowsweet, Calendula, Glycerin, Aloe Vera Gel, Alpha Hydroxy Acid Complex (Citric Acid, Lactic Acid, Malic Acid), Avocado Oil, Sesame Oil, Algae Extract, Panthenol (Pro-Vitamin B5), Green Tea Extract, Retinyl Palmitate (Vitamin A), Ascorbic Acid (Vitamin C), Tocopherol (Vitamin E)
Murad Moisturizing Acne Treatment Gel	Treatment Oily/Acne	Salicylic Acid, Glycerin, Panthenol, Bisabolol (Chamomile), Retinol, Phospholipids, Tocopheryl Acetate (Vitamin E), Retinyl Palmitate (Vitamin A), Dipotassium Glycyrrhizate (Licorice Extract), Farnesol, Lavandula Angustifolia (Lavender) Oil

Product	Type	Ingredients
Joey New York Pure Pores Blackhead Remover and Pore Minimizer Gel	Treatment Oily/Acne	Salicylic Acid, Aloe Extract, AHA (Fruit Acid), Allantoin, Hops Extract, Vitamin E Acetate
Origins Matte Scientist	Treatment Oily/Acne	Chamomile, Sodium Hyaluronate, Salicylic Acid, Tocopheryl Acetate, Linoleic Acid, Green Tea Extract, Phospholipids
Murad Night Reform Treatment	Anti-aging Treatment	Glycolic Acid, Zinc Aspartate, Retinyl Palmitate (Vitamin A), Tocopherol (Vitamin E), Magnesium Ascorbyl Phosphate (Vitamin C), Dipotassium Glycyrrhizate (Licorice Extract), Vitis Vinifera (Grape) Seed Extract, Glycolipids, Hyaluronic Acid, Allantoin
Alba Botanica Beta-Z Night Time Renewal, All Skin Types	Anti-aging Treatment	Chamomile, Glycerin, Aloe Vera, Salicylic Acid, Hyaluronic Acid, Beta Glucan (Oat), Ascorbic Acid (Vitamin C), Licorice Root Extract
Estée Lauder Diminish Anti-Wrinkle Treatment	Anti-aging Treatment	Retinol, Shea Butter, Sodium Hyaluronate, Green Tea Extract, Oat Extract, Tocopheryl Acetate (Vitamin E), Magnesium Ascorbyl Phosphate (Vitamin C), Soybean Oil, Lavender

All of the products mentioned in this chart contain a hydrator, an antioxidant, and a skin soother. In some cases, they also contain additional active ingredients. The Murad product appears first, and other products follow. Since formulas and sources of ingredients vary widely, the effectiveness, safety, and cosmetic considerations may vary from one product to another. Also, in some people, using different brands of products may cause interactions that are unpredictable.

Product Name	Product Category	Hydrating, Antioxidant and Skin Soothing Ingredients
Murad Brightening Treatment SPF 15	Skin Brightening Treatment	Uva Ursi Leaf Extract, Mitracarpus Scaber Extract, Licorice (Glycyrrhiza Glabra) Extract, Mulberry (Morus Nigra) Root Extract, Green Tea (Camellia Sinensis) Extract, Zinc Aspartate, Sodium Hyaluronate Bisabolol, Glycerin
DDF Intensive Holistic Lightener	Skin Brightening Treatment	Glycolic Acid, Kojic Acid, Licorice Extract, Mulberry Extract, Green Tea Extract, Vitamin C
Skin Ceuticals Phyto Corrective Gel	Skin Brightening Treatment	Uva Ursi Extract, Sodium Hyaluronate, Cucumber Extract, Bioflavonoids
Murad Age Spot and Pigment Lightening Gel	Pigmentation Treatment	Hydroquinone (2%), Glycolic Acid, Aloe Barbadenis Leaf Juice, Glycerin, Zinc Aspartate, Tocopherol (Vitamin E), Magnesium Ascorbyl Phosphate (Vitamin C), Dipotassium Glycyrrhizate (Licorice Extract), Vitis Vinifera (Grape) Seed Extract, Allantoin
Philosophy A Pigment of Your Imagination	Pigmentation Treatment	Hydroquinone, Salicylic Acid, Glycerin, Kojic Acid, Lemon Extract, Cucumber Extract, Tocopherol (Vitamin E), Ascorbyl Palmitate, Ascorbic Acid (Vitamin C), Aloe Barbadensis Gel, Sorbitol, Panthenol

Product	Treatment	Ingredients
Peter Thomas Roth Potent Skin Lightening Lotion Complex	Pigmentation Treatment	Hydroquinone (2%), Glycolic Acid, Glycerin, Ascorbic Acid, Vitamins A & E, Licorice Root Extract
Murad Essential-C Eye Cream SPF 15	Eye Treatment Morning	Zinc Aspartate, Retinol, Glycine, Soja (Soybean) Oil, Persea Gratissima (Avocado) Oil, Ascorbyl Palmitate (Vitamin C), Cimicifuga Racemosa Root Extract, Caffeine, Centella Asiatica Extract, Phospholipids, Tocopheryl Acetate (Vitamin E), Retinyl Palmitate, Panthenol, Sodium PCA
Osmotics Daily Eye Protection SPF 15	Eye Treatment Morning	Aloe Vera, Glycerin, Tocopherol Acetate (Vitamin E), Retinyl Palmitate (Vitamin A), Sodium PCA, Avocado Oil, Evening Primrose Oil, Shea Butter
Murad Eye Treatment Complex SPF 8	Eye Treatment Evening	Glycolic Acid, Glycerin, Vitis Vinifera (Grape) Seed Extract, Glycolipids, Zinc Aspartate, Hyaluronic Acid, Tocopherol (Vitamin E), Magnesium Ascorbyl Phosphate (Vitamin C), Dipotassium Glycyrrhizate (Licorice Extract), Retinyl Palmitate (Vitamin A), Panthenol, Allantoin

All of the products mentioned in this chart contain a hydrator, an antioxidant, and a skin soother. In some cases, they also contain additional active ingredients. The Murad product appears first, and other products follow. Since formulas and sources of ingredients vary widely, the effectiveness, safety, and cosmetic considerations may vary from one product to another. Also, in some people, using different brands of products may cause interactions that are unpredictable.

Product Name	Product Category	Hydrating, Antioxidant and Skin Soothing Ingredients
Bobbi Brown Hydrating Eye Cream	Eye Treatment	Glycerin, Cucumber Extract, Green Tea Extract, Magesium Ascorbyl Phosphate, Tocopheryl Acetate, Sodium Hyaluronate, Retinyl Palmitate
Hope Aesthetics BHW Intensive Hydrating Eye Gel	Eye Treatment	Aloe Vera, Cucumber Extract, Glycerin, Evening Primrose, Sodium Hyaluronate, Tocopheryl Acetate (Vitamin E), Retinyl (Vitamin A), Ascorbyl Acetate (Vitamin C), Allantoin, Panthenol (Vitamin B5)
Murad Vitamin C Infusion System	Weekly Vitamin C Treatment	Ascorbic Acid (Vitamin C), Amino Acids, Glycerin, Retinyl Palmitate (Vitamin A), Beta-Carotene, Ranunculus Ficaria (Pilewort) Extract, Zinc Aspartate
Philosophy Hope and a Prayer	Weekly Vitamin C Treatment	Ascorbic Acid, Panthenol, Zinc, Aloe Barbadensis Gel, Algae Extract, Tocopheryl Acetate, Camellia Oleifera Extract (Green Tea), Dipotassium Glycyrrhizate (Licorice), Ascorbyl Palmitate (Vitamin C)
Murad Exfoliating Fruit Enzyme Mask	Exfoliating Mask	Cirtus Medica Limoun (Lemon) Fruit Extract, Bromelain (Pineapple), Ginkgo Biloba Leaf Extract, Glycerin, Carica Papaya (Papaya) Fruit Extract, Lavendula Angustifolia (Lavender) Oil

Product	Type	Ingredients
Astara Violet Flame Purification Mask	Exfoliating Mask	Chamomile, Rosemary, Comfrey, Glycerin, Aloe Vera Gel, Papaya Extract, Papain (Papaya Enzymes), Retinyl Palmitate (Vitamin A), Ascorbic Acid (Vitamin C)
Murad Cellular Replenishing Serum	Hydrating Serum Oily	Glycerin, Glycolipids, Hyaluronic Acid, Anthemis Nobilis (Chamomile) Flower Extract, Tocopherol (Vitamin E), Magnesium Ascorbyl Phosphate (Vitamin C), Vitis Vinifera (Grape) Seed Extract, Camellia Oleifera Leaf (Green Tea) Extract, Cucumis Sativus (Cucumber) Fruit Extract, Arnica Montana Flower Extract
Dior NoAge Defense Renewal Serum	Hydrating Serum Oily	Glycerin, Tocopherol Acetate, Sodium Hyaluronate, Ginseng Root Extract
DDF Cellular Revitalization Age Renewal	Hydrating Serum Oily	Glycerin, Oenothera Biennis (Evening Primrose) Oil, Borago Officinalis Seed Oil, Panthenol, Retinyl Palmitate (Vitamin A)

All of the products mentioned in this chart contain a hydrator, an antioxidant, and a skin soother. In some cases, they also contain additional active ingredients. The Murad product appears first, and other products follow. Since formulas and sources of ingredients vary widely; the effectiveness, safety, and cosmetic considerations may vary from one product to another. Also, in some people, using different brands of products may cause interactions that are unpredictable.

Product Name	Product Category	Hydrating, Antioxidant and Skin Soothing Ingredients
Murad Skin Perfecting Lotion	Hydrating Lotion Normal/Oily	Glycerin, Retinol, Arnica Montana Extract, Vitis Vinifera (Grape) Seed Extract, Camellia Sinesis (Green Tea) Leaf Extract, Spiraea Ulmaria Extract (Meadowsweet), Hyaluronic Acid, Panthenol, Tocopherol (Vitamin E), Magnesium Ascorbyl Phosphate (Vitamin C), Algae Extract, Sodium PCA
Philosophy Help Me	Hydrating Lotion Normal/Oily	Glycerin, Retinol, Tocopherol Acetate, Ascorbyl Palmitate, Bisabolol
St. Ives Hypo-Allergenic Oil-Free Facial Moisturizer	Hydrating Lotion Normal/Oily	Glycerin, Tocopherol Acetate, Retinyl Palmitate, Ascorbic Acid, Aloe Barbadensis Gel, Allantoin, Sodium PCA, Panthenol, Sodium Hyaluronate
Murad Perfecting Day Cream SPF 15	Hydrate Morning Dry	Glycerin, Citrus Medica Limonum (Lemon) Peel Extract, Calendula Extract, Glycolipids, Hyaluronic Acid, Tocopherol (Vitamin E), Magnesium Ascorbyl Phosphate (Vitamin C), Vitis Vinifera (Grape) Seed Extract, Camellia Sinesis (Green Tea), Oenothera Biennis (Evening Primrose) Oil, Borago Officinalis Seed Oil, Sodium PCA
Beauty Without Cruelty SPF 15 Daily Facial Lotion	Hydrate Morning Dry	Green Tea, Vitamin C, Chamomile, Rosemary, Sage, Glycerin, Tocopherol (Vitamin E), Borage Oil, Vitamin A, Allantoin

Product	Timing	Skin Type	Ingredients
Elizabeth Arden Ceramide Time Complex Moisture Cream, SPF 15	Hydrate Morning	Dry	Glycerin, Sphingolipids, Sodium Hyaluronate, Sodium PCA, Ascorbyl Palmitate, Tocopheryl Acetate, Glycine, Serine
Murad Perfecting Night Cream	Hydrate Evening	Dry	Helianthus Annuus (Hybrid Sunflower) Oil, Glycerin, Algae Extract, Borogo Officinalis Seed Oil, Oenothera Biennis (Evening Primrose) Oil, Panthenol, Vitis Vinifera (Grape) Seed Extract, Camellia Sinensis (Green Tea) Leaf Extract, Tocopherol (Vitamin E), Magnesium Ascorbyl Phosphate, Retinyl Palmitate (Vitamin A), Glycolipids, Hyaluronic Acid
Ecco Bella Skin Survival Night Cream with Ceramide 3	Hydrate Evening	Dry	Sunflower Oil, Jojoba Oil, Vitamin E, Ascorbyl Palmitate (Vitamin C), Oat Flour, Sodium Hyaluronate, Calendula, Chamomile, Arnica, Grapefruit Seed Extract, Lavender
Osmotics Intensive Moisture Therapy	Hydrate Evening	Dry	Aloe Vera, Glycerin, Sunflower Seed Oil, Sodium PCA, Vitamin E Extract, Ascorbic Acid, Evening Primrose Oil, Betaglucan, Avocado Oil, Retinyl Palmitate (Vitamin A)

All of the products mentioned in this chart contain a hydrator, an antioxidant, and a skin soother. In some cases, they also contain additional active ingredients. The Murad product appears first, and other products follow. Since formulas and sources of ingredients vary widely, the effectiveness, safety, and cosmetic considerations may vary from one product to another. Also, in some people, using different brands of products may cause interactions that are unpredictable.

Product Name	Product Category	Hydrating, Antioxidant and Skin Soothing Ingredients
Astara Antioxidant Light Moisturizer	Hydrate Evening Dry	Aloe Vera Gel, Sodium Hyaluronate, Borage Oil, Vitamin E Linoleate, Vitamin E Acetate, Beta Glucan, Green Tea Extract, Panthenol, Sodium PCA, Ascorbic Acid (Vitamin C), (Vitamin E) Grape Seed Extract, Sodium PCA
Murad Exfoliating Acne Treatment Gel	Treatment Acne Concern	Glycolic Acid, Salicylic Acid, Aloe Barbadensis Leaf Extract, Rice Amino Acids, Zinc Aspartate, Retinol (Vitamin A), Arnica Montanta Flower Extract, Tocopherol (Vitamin E), Magnesium Ascorbyl Phosphate (Vitamin C), Dipotassium Glycyrrhizate (Licorice Extract), Vitis Vinifera (Grape) Seed Extract, Camellia Sinensis (Green Tea) Leaf Extract, Zinc Acetate
Neutrogena Skin Clearing Moisturizer Face Cream with Salicylic Acid & Retinol	Treatment Acne Concern	Salicylic Acid, Allantoin, Glycerin, Piper Methysticum (Kawa) Extract, Panthenol, Retinol, Tocopherol
Phytomer Acnigel	Treatment Acne Concern	Orris Extract, Zinc PCA, Retinyl Palmitate, Hazelnut Oil, Glycerin, Corallina Officinalis Extract, Tocopherol Linoleate

Product	Type	Ingredients
Murad Acne Spot Treatment	Acne Spot Treatment	Glycolic Acid, Zinc Oxide, Citrus Autantium Dulcis (Orange Oil), Salicylic Acid, Tocopherol, (Vitamin E), Magnesium Ascorbyl Phosphate (Vitamin C), Dipotassium Glycyrrhizate (Licorice Extract) Vitis Vinifera (Grape) Seed Extract, Allantoin
Neova Intensive Blemish Treatment	Acne Spot Treatment	Algae Extract, Glycerin, Salicylic Acid, Betaglucan, Camellia Oleifera Extract, Diptassium Glycyrrhizinate, Dydrocohyl, Asiatica Extract, Coneflower Extract, Tea Tree Oil, Eucalyptus Oil, Wild Thyme Oil, Sage Oil
Murad Perfecting Serum	Hydrating Serum Dry	Ceramides, Sphingolipids, Tocopheryl Acetate (Vitamin E), Evening Primrose Oil, Avocado Oil, Retinyl Palmitate (Vitamin A), Squalane (Olives)
Emulsion d'Olives	Hydrating Serum Dry	Olea Europaea (Olive) Oil Unsaponifiables, Cannabis Sativa Seed Oil, Shorea Stenoptera Butter, Olea Europaea (Olive) Leaf Extract, Glycine Soja (Soybean) Oil, Sodium Hyaluronate, Tocopheryl Acetate, Allantoin, Bisabolol, Linoleic Acid, Retinyl Palmitate, Tocopherol, Zinc PCA

All of the products mentioned in this chart contain a hydrator, an antioxidant, and a skin soother. In some cases, they also contain additional active ingredients. The Murad product appears first, and other products follow. Since formulas and sources of ingredients vary widely, the effectiveness, safety, and cosmetic considerations may vary from one product to another. Also, in some people, using different brands of products may cause interactions that are unpredictable.

Product Name	Product Category	Hydrating, Antioxidant and Skin Soothing Ingredients
Z. Bigatti Re-Storation Deep Repair Facial Serum	Hydrating Serum Dry	Grape Seed Extract, Glycerine, Apricot Kernel Oil, Horse Chestnut Extract, Comfrey Leaf Extract, Cucumber Fruit Extract, Green Tea Extract, Soybean Oil, Tocopheryl Acetate, Linoleic Acid, Lemon Peel Extract, Kelp Extract, Ginseng Root Extract, Lemongrass Extract, Matricaria Extract, Sodium Hyaluronate, Retinyl Palmitate, Arginine, Panthenol
Murad Age-Balancing Night Cream	Hydrate Evening Menopausal Concern	Persea Gratissima (Avocado) Oil, Trifolium Pratense (Clove) Flower Extract, Mendahen Oil, Retinol, Borago Officinalis Seed Oil, Oenothera Biennis (Evening Primrose) Oil, Sodium Ascorbyl Phosphate (Vitamin C), Tocopheryl Acetate (Vitamin E), Sodium PCA, Panthenol, Citrus Aurantium Dulcis (Orange) Oil, Glycine Soja (Soybean) Oil
Murad Oil-Free Sunblock SPF 15	Oil-Free Sunblock SPF 15+	Punica Granatum (Pomegranate) Extract, Zinc Aspartate, Rice Amino Acids, Tocopherol (Vitamin E), Magnesium Ascorbyl Phosphate (Vitamin C), Sodium PCA, Retinyl Palmitate (Vitamin A), Vitis Vinifera (Grape) Seed Extract, Citrus Medica Limonum (Lemon) Peel Extract

Product	Type	Ingredients
Neutrogena Healthy Defense Oil-Free Sunblock Lotion, SPF 45	Oil-Free Sunblock SPF 15+	Glycerin, Tocopheryl Acetate, Retinyl Palmitate, Ascorbyl Palmitate, Bisabolol
Naturopathica Lavender UV Protective Cream	Oil-Free Sunblock SPF 15+	Vitamin A, Vitamin E, Vitamin C, Glycerin, Lavender
Murad Hydrating Sunscreen SPF 15	Hydrating Sunscreen SPF 15+	Punica Granatum (Pomegranate) Extract, Zinc Aspartate, Rice Amino Acids, Tocopherol (Vitamin E), Magnesium Ascorbyl Phosphate (Vitamin C), Sodium PCA, Retinyl Palmitate (Vitamin A), Vitis Vinifera (Grape) Seed Extract, Glycolipids, Hyaluronic Acid, Sodium PCA, Citrus Medica Limonum (Lemon) Peel Extract
Essential Elements Sun Protection Moisturizer, SPF 15, All Skin Types	Hydrating Sunscreen SPF 15+	Aloe Vera, Glycerin, Jojoba Oil, Tocopherol, Green Tea, Hyaluronic Acid, Retinyl Palmitate, Licorice Extract

All of the products mentioned in this chart contain a hydrator, an antioxidant, and a skin soother. In some cases, they also contain additional active ingredients. The Murad product appears first, and other products follow. Since formulas and sources of ingredients vary widely, the effectiveness, safety, and cosmetic considerations may vary from one product to another. Also, in some people, using different brands of products may cause interactions that are unpredictable.

Product Name	Product Category	Hydrating, Antioxidant and Skin Soothing Ingredients
Murad Waterproof Sunblock SPF 30	Waterproof Sunblock SPF 15+	Punica Granatum (Pomegranate) Extract, Zinc Aspartate, Rice Amino Acids, Tocopherol (Vitamin E), Magnesium Ascorbyl Phosphate (Vitamin C), Sodium PCA, Retinyl Palmitate (Vitamin A), Vitis Vinifera (Grape) Seed Extract, Glycolipids, Hyaluronic Acid, Citrus Medica Limonum (Lemon) Peel Extract
Osmotics Protection Extreme for Face and Body SPF 25	Waterproof Sunblock SPF 15+	Corn Oil, Squalane, Grape Seed Extract, Retinyl Palmitate (Vitamin A)
DDF Sport Proof SPF 30	Waterproof Sunblock SPF 15+	Vitamin A, Vitamin C, Vitamin E, Zinc, Grape Seed Extract

All of the products mentioned in this chart contain a hydrator, an antioxidant, and a skin soother. In some cases, they also contain additional active ingredients. The Murad product appears first, and other products follow. Since formulas and sources of ingredients vary widely, the effectiveness, safety, and cosmetic considerations may vary from one product to another. Also, in some people, using different brands of products may cause interactions that are unpredictable.

Index

Acknowledgments

This book took more than a year to complete, but it was years in the making. Each time I've lectured at medical and esthetician conferences, discussed my program with fellow physicians, and been interviewed by journalists, I've thought to myself, "I need to write about my program." In 1999, my friend and publicist, Harris Shepard, refused to let me procrastinate any longer and introduced me to my coauthor saying, "Let's do it."

We have many people to thank. At the top of our list is Lisa Polley, director of Corporate Communications for Murad, Inc., who was always willing to talk about concepts, review drafts, and muster resources. We are grateful to our agent, Barbara Lowenstein of Lowenstein-Yost Associates. We thank Elizabeth Beier for her clear direction and her editorial savvy. We are grateful to the many patients and estheticians who shared their experiences with us.

On a personal level, I will forever be grateful to my parents, Rachel and Albert Murad, who immigrated to this country with six children, including six-year-old me. Because of my parents' bravery and sacrifice I was fortunate to grow up and live in a society that gave me the opportunity to fulfill my dreams.

I would also like to thank my large extended family and especially my children, Hilarie, Elizabeth, and Jeff, for their love and support. And I thank my dearest friend, Loralee Knotts, whose optimism, caring, and honesty have added so much to my life.

—*Howard Murad, M.D.*

I would like to remember and thank my mentor and friend Phyllis Starr Wilson, the founding editor of *Self* magazine. I'm grateful to my son, Jordan Partie, who has never complained when deadlines took priority, and to my best friend, Marvin Jacoby, whose patience never falters.

—*Dianne Partie Lange*

RECEIVE A SPECIAL OFFER FROM DR. MURAD, HERE'S HOW:

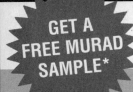

GET A FREE MURAD SAMPLE*

1. Log on to www.murad.com/consultation
2. Answer a few questions about your skin and lifestyle
3. Receive your personalized Murad Method skincare prescription for Wrinkle-Free Skin
4. Learn how to receive your FREE product*

Or call **1-800-33MURAD** to speak to a trained Murad Skincare Consultant

*Offer valid only while supplies last or until July 1, 2005. You must be a legal resident of the U.S. or Canada and 18 years or older to be eligible. No purchase necessary. Void where prohibited.

Murad.® Where skincare meets healthcare